100 Questions & Answers About Arthritis

Campion Quinn, MD, MHA

Long Island, New York

Larry Greenbaum, MD

Indiana Internal Medicine Consultants
Greenwood, Indiana

JONES AND BARTLETT PUBLISHERS

Sudbury, Massachusetts

BOSTON   TORONTO   LONDON   SINGAPORE

World Headquarters
Jones and Bartlett Publishers
40 Tall Pine Drive
Sudbury, MA 01776
978-443-5000
info@jbpub.com
www.jbpub.com

Jones and Bartlett Publishers
Canada
6339 Ormindale Way
Mississauga, Ontario L5V 1J2
CANADA

Jones and Bartlett Publishers
International
Barb House, Barb Mews
London W6 7PA
UK

Jones and Bartlett's books and products are available through most bookstores and online booksellers. To contact Jones and Bartlett Publishers directly, call 800-832-0034, fax 978-443-8000, or visit our website, www.jbpub.com.

Substantial discounts on bulk quantities of Jones and Bartlett's publications are available to corporations, professional associations, and other qualified organizations. For details and specific discount information, contact the special sales department at Jones and Bartlett via the above contact information or send an email to specialsales@jbpub.com.

Production Credits
Executive Publisher: Christopher Davis
Associate Editor: Kathy Richardson
Production Director: Amy Rose
Associate Production Editor: Rachel Rossi
Associate Marketing Manager: Rebecca Wasley

Manufacturing Buyer: Therese Connell
Cover Design: Jon Ayotte
Composition: Appingo
Printing and Binding: Malloy, Inc.
Cover Printing: Malloy, Inc.

Library of Congress Cataloging-in-Publication Data
Quinn, Campion.
  100 questions and answers about arthritis / Campion Quinn.
    p. cm.
  Includes index.
  ISBN-13: 978-0-7637-4051-1 (pbk. : alk. paper)
  ISBN-10: 0-7637-4051-9
  1. Arthritis--Miscellanea. 2. Arthritis--Popular works. I. Title. II. Title: One hundred questions and answers about arthritis.
  RC933.Q85 2008
  616.7'22--dc22
                            2007021401
6048

Printed in the United States of America
11 10 09 08 07 10 9 8 7 6 5 4 3 2 1

This book is dedicated to all those people who suffer from the devastating effects of arthritis and for those doctors who care for them.

CONTENTS

Part 1: Rheumatoid Arthritis: the Basics   1

Questions 1-10 cover background information about rheumatoid arthrisis, including:

- What is rheumatoid arthritis?
- Is rheumatoid arthritis serious?
- Is rheumatoid arthritis a genetic disease?

Part 2: My Rheumatoid Arthritis Treatment Team   19

Questions 11-16 discuss various professionals that you may come across in your treatment and dealings with rheumatoid arthritis, such as:

- What type of doctor should I see for my rheumatoid arthritis?
- Is there a difference between a medical intern and a rheumatologist?
- What is an occupational therapist, and why does my doctor want me to see one?

Part 3: Rheumatoid Arthritis: Not Just a Disease of the Joints   33

Questions 17-30 describe symptoms of rheumatoid arthritis that reach beyond your joints, such as:

- My rheumatoid arthritis makes me very tired. Is that normal?
- Will my rheumatoid arthritis affect the eyes?
- Can my rheumatoid arthritis cause a low blood count?

Part 4: Treatment of Rheumatoid Arthritis: General Principles   61

Questions 31-35 are concerned with general questions:

- How will my doctor choose the right medication for me?
- I've had rheumatoid arthritis for a long time. Is it too late to treat it?
- Can rheumatoid arthritis be put into remission?

Contents

Part 10: Treatment for Osteoarthritis   *165*

Questions 79-100 address both traditional and alternative treatment options for osteoarthritis, including:

- Does glucosamine and chondroitin sulfate work for osteoarthritis?
- Can the osteoporosis drug, risedronate, help treat osteoarthritis?
- Is joint replacement an option for the treatment of osteoarthritis symptoms?

INTRODUCTION

This book was written for people with arthritis and their families. It covers the two most common types of arthritis: rheumatoid arthritis and osteo-arthritis. It is the hope of the authors that this book can provide useful information about arthritis and that this information will help the people live healthier and more comfortable lives.

Although this book can be read from cover to cover, it was designed as a reference text, so that an arthritis sufferer or his or her caregiver can review sections whose information is of immediate importance.

This book is not a comprehensive discussion of arthritis. The authors chose to address the questions about this disease that are most frequently asked, in order to explore them in as much detail as possible.

Nona's Biography

I am 53 years old now and was diagnosed with rheumatoid arthritis about 14 years ago. These were the early years of my marriage and I was pregnant with my second child. Although at times it's been a struggle trying to control the progression of my disease, I have remained extremely active and have not let it interfere with the activities I love: skiing, tennis, gardening, hiking—in general, a very active outdoor lifestyle with my husband and two children. At this point in my life, I am looking very positively toward the future.

Jim's Biography

I am a 68-year-old man who has had rheumatoid arthritis for approximately 35 years. I was diagnosed in 1972. For the first three years I was on all types of RA meds. In 1975, we went with the gold treatment, one injection once a week to one injection once a month. In 1993, with the anti-inflammatory drug prednisone, the gold shots ended. Also in 1993 we went to methotrexate—six 2.5 mg tabs once a week with prednisone, plaquenil, and folic acid daily. Prednisone was discontinued in 1994. Currently I am on 4 methotrexate a week, but have been on as few as three a week. The change in seasons often causes my arthritis to flare up. Sometimes I require a change in my medications to reduce the pain and bring my disease back under control.

PART ONE

Rheumatoid Arthritis: The Basics

What is rheumatoid arthritis?

What are the symptoms of rheumatoid arthritis?

Is rheumatoid arthritis serious?

More . . .

1. What is rheumatoid arthritis?

The ancient Greeks were aware that joint and muscle aches were sometimes associated with colds. The word *rheuma* in Greek means "flow" or "discharge," where this "flow" refers to the watery discharge from the eyes and nose during a cold. The word **arthritis** is also derived from the Greek—specifically, from *arthron* (or **arthr-**), meaning "joint," and **itis,** meaning "inflammation." Thus **rheumatoid arthritis (RA)** was originally thought to be a disease that resulted in painful and swollen joints and that was caused by a cold.

Today, RA is still a description for a medical condition that is characterized by painful inflamed joints, but the association with watery eyes and runny noses has been discarded by modern physicians. RA is currently understood to be a **systemic** inflammatory disease that affects the joints and other tissues in the body. It is both **chronic** and **progressive**.

When doctors describe rheumatoid arthritis as a chronic illness, they mean that it can last for years. In some patients, disease activity may be characterized by frequent **flares**. Other patients may go for long periods without any symptoms at all. For the majority of patients, however, RA symptoms are something they deal with every day. This disease is progressive in nature, meaning that it tends to get worse over time. RA also has the potential to cause chronic pain, joint destruction, and functional disability.

RA affects the joints by causing an **inflammation** of the specialized cells that cover the ends of bones and line the joint. These specialized cells are collectively called the **synovium**. The inflammation in RA is caused by a person's own immune system attacking his or her own body's tissues. This type of reaction is called an "autoimmune" reaction; hence RA is sometimes referred to as an **autoimmune disease.**

RA affects 1% of the U.S. population, or approximately 2.1 million Americans. Currently, its cause is unknown, although

Arthritis

Inflammation of a joint, usually accompanied by pain, swelling, and stiffness.

Arthr-

A prefix meaning "joint."

Rheumatoid arthritis (RA)

A chronic autoimmune disease characterized by pain, stiffness, inflammation, swelling, and sometimes destruction of joints.

Systemic

An adjective used in medicine to indicate something that affects the entire body, rather than a single part or organ.

Chronic

Lasting for a long time. The word comes from the Greek *chronos,* which means "time."

Progressive

An adjective applied to many diseases; it suggests an increase in scope or severity of disease.

several theories have been suggested regarding its origins. For example, scientists hypothesize that RA may be caused by a complex interaction between a person's genetic makeup and his or her environment.

2. What are the symptoms of rheumatoid arthritis?

More than 200 types of arthritis have been identified. One way that physicians distinguish one type of arthritis from another is by its characteristic location, physical findings, laboratory tests, and x-rays. Early on in the disease, making a **diagnosis** of RA can be difficult for your physician because your symptoms may change over time. The "classic symptoms" of RA are pain, swelling, stiffness, fatigue, weight loss, and joint deformity. A patient may have all of these symptoms or just a few. The symptoms may be severe and disabling or merely annoying. During the course of the disease, new symptoms can appear and others may disappear with treatment.

The main symptom of RA is joint stiffness. This stiffness occurs primarily in the hands or feet and affects the small joints first. When more than one joint is affected, the swelling is symmetrical. That is, the swelling tends to affect the same joints in both the right and left sides of the body at the same time. This condition is generally observed in RA that has been present for a few months or longer. Very early RA may not always be symmetrical, however, which increases the difficulty of making the correct diagnosis. The swelling is usually worse in the morning and improves by midday. Stiffness that persists for an hour or more, or swelling and pain that last for more than six weeks, may also be indicative of RA.

In this disease, the lining of the joint, called the synovium, is attacked by **antibodies** and white blood cells. This attack causes inflammation, redness, and swelling of the joint. The joint can become exquisitely tender, making even small movements impossible. Like the stiffness associated with RA, this

Flare

The reappearance or worsening of arthritic symptoms.

Inflammation

A response to injury or foreign invasion that is designed to protect the body. Its symptoms include heat, redness, swelling, and pain.

Autoimmune disease

A disease that arises when an individual's immune system reacts against his or her own organs and tissues.

The main symptom of RA is joint stiffness; persistent joint pain is another symptom commonly associated with RA.

Diagnosis

The identification of an illness after review of the patient's clinical history, physical exam, and laboratory tests.

Rheumatoid Arthritis: The Basics

Antibodies

Proteins produced by white blood cells to fight foreign proteins, viruses, bacteria, and other unfamiliar invaders.

Range of motion (ROM)

Measurement of joint movement angle, which may be restricted due to inflammation.

Erosion

From the Latin *erodere,* meaning "to eat away"; an eating away of a surface. Erosion of the bone surface of joints is a common feature of many types of arthritis.

Crepitus

A crackling sound or grating sensation in a joint, caused by swollen synovium or bone surface rubbing together.

joint pain tends to be symmetrical, although sometimes a single swollen painful joint is the presenting symptom of RA. The joint pain in RA is aggravated by movement or activity, such as walking, getting up from a chair, carrying groceries, or just getting dressed.

The pain and stiffness of RA often lead to a decreased **range of motion** in the affected joints. Range of motion (which is often abbreviated as ROM in physicians' notes) is the extent to which a joint can be flexed or extended naturally. Thus a restricted or limited range of motion is a reduction in a joint's normal range of movement. RA can cause a limited range of motion by producing joint swelling, bone **erosion,** or tissue impingement. Having a limited range of motion can prevent you from getting a can off a high shelf, brushing your hair, or putting on your shoes.

Long-standing RA may lead to joint deformity. That is, the chronic inflammation of RA can cause loss of cartilage and bone in the joint. The loss of these tissues may, in turn, cause the joint to become unstable and dysfunctional. As a consequence of these changes, your physician may notice a symptom called **crepitus** when he or she moves your joint. Crepitus is a crackling, grinding, or grating feeling or sound in the joints when they are flexed and extended. Joint crepitus is associated with significant cartilage loss and joint destruction.

In the past, joint deformity and joint destruction were typical outcomes with long-standing RA. Now, however, thanks to newer therapies that are applied earlier, there is a dramatic decrease in the amount of joint deformity and destruction experienced by people with RA.

Not all of the symptoms of RA are associated with the joints. Early-stage RA may produce systemic symptoms such as fever, chills, excessive tiredness, or rash. Small pea-sized lumps called **rheumatoid nodules** may also develop in the skin. Some patients experience a loss of appetite that can result in significant weight loss. **Anemia** (that is, a low red blood cell count) is another common finding in patients with RA.

When I look back now, although I didn't realize it at the time, the first signs of my arthritis started about 17 years ago while playing tennis. It just seemed like it would take forever to warm up. My hands and wrist were weak and finally I could hardly hold the racquet. At the time, I got really frustrated, blamed it on my lack of ability and just quit playing. The next time it was an issue was a few years later when I was pregnant with my second child. My hands got so swollen that I couldn't tie my shoes or even manage to change a diaper. I still didn't attribute this to arthritis, but rather to swelling caused by my pregnancy. Finally, I started to have severe pain in my feet. I could hardly get out of bed because it was so painful to put pressure on the balls of my feet. This is when I saw my family doctor and he immediately referred me to a rheumatologist.

—Nona

3. Is rheumatoid arthritis serious?

Yes, RA is a serious disease. While some people suffer only mild discomfort and minimal disability, medical studies have demonstrated that one third of patients are unable to work five years after they are diagnosed. At ten years, more than half of all people with RA are unable to work.

Daily joint pain is an inevitable consequence of this disease. Affected joints can become deformed, and the performance of even ordinary tasks may be very difficult or impossible. In one survey of patients with RA, 70% indicated that the disease prevented them from living a fully productive life. Respondents to that survey reported that RA interfered with their ability to carry out normal daily activities, limited their job opportunities, and decreased the joys and responsibilities of family life. Most patients also experienced some degree of depression, anxiety, and feelings of helplessness.

Rheumatoid nodules

Firm, nonpainful lumps in the skin of patients with rheumatoid arthritis. These nodules tend to occur at pressure points of the body—most commonly, the elbows. They are a sign of long-standing rheumatoid arthritis.

Anemia

The condition of having less than the normal number of red blood cells or less than the normal quantity of hemoglobin in the blood. Anemia is associated with rheumatoid arthritis and other chronic diseases. It a complication of the use of nonsteroidal anti-inflammatory drugs (NSAIDs).

Rheumatoid Arthritis: The Basics

The effects of RA are not just limited to joint pain and stiffness. This disease can affect many organs in the body. It can cause skin lesions, lung fibrosis, **osteoporosis**, eye inflammation, and blindness. Severe infections, gastrointestinal (GI) problems, low blood counts, and some types of cancers and **lymphomas** are all more common in patients with RA than in the general public. Similarly, diseases of the teeth and gums are more common in these patients. People with RA may be twice as likely as non-arthritic individuals to have periodontal diseases: Chronic inflammation and immune dysfunction are central characteristics of these diseases. Recent research indicates that people with RA—and particularly those whose disease is not well controlled—may have a higher risk for heart disease and stroke. While RA is not fatal, its complications may shorten the life span of affected individuals to a significant extent.

From an economic standpoint, the costs of medical and surgical treatment, plus the expense of lost wages due to disability caused by RA, add up to millions of dollars.

Although RA is a serious disease, it is not a reason for despair. With early, aggressive treatment, the symptoms can be improved and disability can be lessened or eliminated completely.

I'll never forget that day when my doctor confirmed the diagnosis and told me that I had rheumatoid arthritis. My reaction was shock and disbelief. Sure I had all these symptoms and my hands kept swelling but I thought it had to be a temporary condition. After all, I was only 40 years young with two small children. Arthritis? How can that be? I thought it was a condition that happened to older people. I didn't want to believe it. Since that time I've tried many medications, had a lot of pain and swelling in my hands to the point where I felt handicapped for short periods, but today thanks to new drugs I seldom feel that I even have arthritis.

—Nona

Osteoporosis

A disease characterized by the thinning of the bones with a reduction in bone mass owing to depletion of calcium and bone protein. Osteoporosis predisposes a person to fractures.

Lymphoma

A cancer of the lymphoid tissue.

Although RA is a serious disease; it is not a reason for despair. With early, aggressive treatment, the symptoms can be improved and disability can be lessened or eliminated completely.

4. What causes rheumatoid arthritis?

Despite years of research and study, the precise cause of RA is not known. Physicians have determined that the pain, stiffness, and inflammation associated with this disease result from a disorder in the body's immune system. For unexplained reasons, the body's immune system—in the form of white blood cells and antibodies—attacks the joints and other tissues in the body. The continuous inflammation in the joints accounts for the damage of joints. What triggers this abnormal immune response remains unknown, although genetic factors and infectious/environmental agents have been the targets of the most study.

Genetic Factors

There appears to be a genetic component to RA. Nevertheless, although medical studies suggest that a person's genetic makeup is an important part of the story, it is not the whole answer.

For example, scientists have found that certain genes that play a role in the immune system are associated with a tendency to develop RA. The genes that influence this tendency are more common in the families of people who have RA. Although this "genetic tendency" to develop RA may be passed on to the next generation, the disease does not automatically occur in everyone who inherits the genes. At the same time, some people with RA do not have these particular genes. It is possible that the disease occurs only in people who have a genetic or inherited tendency toward the disease and who are also exposed to other "RA-causing agents."

Environmental Factors

What causes an otherwise healthy person to develop RA? What triggers the immune system to attack the body? Many rheumatologists believe that an infectious agent is the trigger that produces RA in individuals who have an underlying genetic susceptibility to the disease. An infectious agent such as a virus or bacterium may be responsible, but the exact agent is not yet known, despite exhaustive studies.

Other Causes

Why does RA occur more frequently in women than in men? Why does RA occur more frequently in adults than in children? Could hormones have some effect on the development of RA? Some scientists think so. They suggest that hormones, or possibly deficiencies or changes in certain hormones, may promote the development of RA in a person with "RA-prone genes" who has been exposed to a triggering agent from the environment.

After decades of study, scientists don't have all the answers about what causes RA, though most believe that RA develops as a result of an interaction of many factors. In addition to identifying possible causes of this disease, researchers have been able to exclude certain agents as causes of RA. According to scientific evidence now available, RA is *not caused* by any of the following factors:

- Environments that are cold and damp
- Changes in weather or ambient air pressure
- Diet—especially a lack (or excess) of vitamins or any other dietary elements such as fats, sugars, acids, or metals
- Exposure to mercury, arsenic, or other heavy metals
- Faulty absorption or elimination of substances from the bowel
- Infections in the internal organs of the body
- Exposure to radiation or magnetic fields
- The effects of mold or yeast in the environment or in the blood

If you have further questions regarding the causes of RA, discuss them with your rheumatologist, who is an expert in that area.

5. *What is the course of rheumatoid arthritis?*

Rheumatoid arthritis may begin at any age, but the most common age range during which onset begins is the twenties to fifties. Morning stiffness is a hallmark symptom of RA. People with RA often report having a half hour or more of stiffness in the morning. The same symptoms frequently occur after short periods of inactivity such as driving or sitting. For older people, symptoms of weakness or falling may be more common.

For the majority of people, RA begins insidiously, emerging over a period of weeks to months. Typically, a person can only approximately recall when his or her arthritis problems began. Some first notice joint symptoms such as stiffness, joint swelling or pain, puffy hands, or diffuse aches and pains in the muscles. For others, the first problems are systemic symptoms such as fatigue or malaise.

A minority of people with RA experience a sudden onset of severe pain and joint swelling over the course of a few days. Some patients develop their arthritis over an intermediate period of time. Older patients sometimes present with polymyalgia rheumatica (PMR) and progress to RA. PMR is characterized by severe stiffness and aching of the shoulders and hips. I often think of PMR as a limited case of RA. Although PMR is a fairly common disease, only a small percentage of these patients develop RA.

A very few patients have a "palindromic" onset of disease. Palindromic rheumatism is characterized be short, intense episodes of arthritis that typically involve only one or two areas of the body, such as one hand or one foot. These episodes are very painful, but last only a day or two and get better even without treatment. In between episodes, the person is completely free of symptoms or signs of arthritis. This disorder may go on for years, may resolve spontaneously, or may progress into RA or other diseases. It is frequently misdiagnosed as **gout.**

Gout

A disease characterized by increased blood levels of uric acid; it produces pain and inflammation in the joints, particularly in the foot, ankle, and knee.

Rheumatoid Arthritis: The Basics

Early in the course of RA, the small joints of the fingers, wrists, and toes are involved. Large joint involvement typically develops later in the course of the illness. RA is typically a "symmetrical" arthritis, meaning that the right and left sides of the body are affected fairly equally. This is almost always the case in long-standing arthritis, but the symmetry may not be so obvious early in the course of the disease. People with RA sometimes say things such as "Only my right hand is involved," but upon examination a physician will usually find that both hands are affected; the confusion arises because the findings in the other hand may be more subtle and easier to ignore. The dominant hand generally has more severe symptoms, probably because it is used more frequently. Paralysis is a major exception to this general finding. Individuals who are weak or paralyzed on one side of the body, perhaps because of a stroke or other neurological problem, typically have much milder arthritis symptoms on that side, presumably because they no longer use that side of their body very much. Muscle atrophy and weakness around affected joints is a common early finding of RA.

For a fortunate few, RA may spontaneously get better. For the majority of patients who visit arthritis clinics, however, the disease gets worse if it isn't treated in an appropriate and timely fashion. For some patients, severe joint damage can occur within a few years; other individuals may experience a much slower progression of their disease.

People who develop RA early in life tend to have a faster and more severe course. Those who develop their RA later in life tend to have a slower progression of their disease.

As a generalization, people who develop RA early in life have a faster and more severe course. Those who develop their RA later in life tend to have a slower progression of their disease.

If you develop RA symptoms such as joint pain, swelling, and fatigue, you should see your primary care physician as soon as possible. If the diagnosis is uncertain, you should ask for referral to a rheumatologist. Early diagnosis and treatment are the best course of action to minimize the damage that this disease can cause.

It has been quite a roller coaster ride for me these past 17 years; from the initial shock of my diagnosis to finding drugs that work. I've probably tried over 15 different medications. Some would work for a while but then the swelling in my hands would get worse so we would have to try something else. The pain in my feet went away after a very short time and I've never been bothered with that again. I can honestly say that my arthritis has never stopped me from doing any of the activities I love for very long. I am an avid skier, hiker and I'm even playing tennis again. I am responding so well to my medication that I hardly feel I have arthritis. Initially, my flare ups left my hands quite deformed, but now it's really hardly noticeable. It's really now just a little inconvenience that I can certainly live with. Of course, who knows what the future may hold but I've just got to keep on doing everything I love to do now and not worry about what may lie ahead.

—Nona

6. Will I lose the ability to walk?

Untreated RA can cause severe damage to the hips, knees, and feet. However, with current treatments, RA shouldn't progress to the point that you cannot walk. You and your doctor can work together to limit any joint damage and maintain your mobility.

Inability to walk owing to severe RA may involve factors other than RA. Obesity or previous joint damage may lead to secondary osteoarthritis, particularly in the knees. Treatment with **corticosteroids** (prednisone or Medrol) is sometimes necessary to curb the intense inflammation and stiffness associated with RA. Unfortunately, these drugs are a "double-edged sword": They can cause significant weight gain, which in turn contributes to arthritis of the legs. Bacterial joint infection (**septic arthritis**) can also cause severe permanent

Rheumatoid Arthritis: The Basics

Corticosteroids

Any of the steroid hormones made by the cortex (outer layer) of the adrenal gland; also called cortisol and steroids. These potent drugs are used to reduce the pain and inflammation associated with rheumatoid arthritis and other autoimmune disorders.

Septic arthritis

Arthritis caused by invading microorganisms.

joint damage. Fortunately, this is a very infrequent complication of RA.

Chronic treatment with corticosteroids may lead to muscle weakness that can complicate walking-related problems. These medications are also a risk factor for the development of osteoporosis. Falling—or fear of falling—can also dissuade patients from walking. Adaptive devices such as canes, walkers, or Rollators (a rolling walker with a seat) can make a world of difference, although younger patients are sometimes reluctant to use these devices.

Managing RA frequently requires a team approach. For example, your team may include your **rheumatologist,** primary care physician, orthopedic surgeon, rehabilitation specialist (or physiatrist), and physical and occupational therapists. Not everyone needs the care of every member of the treatment team at the same time, of course. As on any team, each member has a specialty that he or she brings to bear as the patient's symptoms dictate.

Rheumatologist

A physician who specializes in the treatment of diseases of the joints and connective tissue.

All patients with a diagnosis of RA should be involved in an exercise program to maintain their strength and flexibility. A physical therapist can help determine your need for therapy and teach you the exercises you should perform every day.

All patients with a diagnosis of RA should be involved in an exercise program to maintain their strength and flexibility.

When joint pain is severe or the range of motion in the joint is limited, consultation with an orthopedic surgeon may be necessary. Hip or knee replacement can create dramatic improvements in the quality of life for patients with severe arthritis of those joints. While orthopedists are skilled in the treatment of severely damaged joints, they should not be solely in charge of the management of a patient with RA. This situation frequently leads to too many surgeries and too little use of disease-modifying drugs.

The worst thing you can do is to ignore your disease. Medical studies have shown that early treatment of RA can halt its progression and reduce the risk that you will suffer permanent joint damage.

7. Will I become disabled and unable to work?

It is impossible to predict the course of RA for a particular person, so it is equally difficult to tell if someone with RA will become disabled. However, the pattern of disease can influence the risk of disability.

For 10% of patients, RA symptoms disappear completely on their own. If disease **remission** occurs, it usually takes place within the first six months after the onset of symptoms. Remissions occur more commonly in those patients who do not have **rheumatoid factor (RF)** in their blood (Question 47 discusses rheumatoid factor). For other individuals, recurrent explosive attacks of joint pain and swelling are followed by periods of little or no symptoms. The most common pattern, however, is one of persistent and progressive disease activity that waxes and wanes in intensity.

Risk factors for disability in RA include the following:

- Long duration of disease
- Many joints involved
- High severity of inflammation of the joints
- Presence of high levels of rheumatoid factor in the blood
- Presence of high levels of cyclic citrullinated peptide (CCP) antibody in the blood (Question 55 discusses CCP antibody)
- High sedimentation rate (Question 26 discusses sedimentation rates)
- Family history of RA

In studies performed before the new therapies became available, approximately one third of patients were disabled after five years and 60% of patients were unable to work after having RA

Remission

A period in the course of a disease during which symptoms of a disease diminish or disappear.

Rheumatoid factor (RF)

An antibody found in about 85% of people with rheumatoid arthritis; it also appears in other diseases and is sometimes found in healthy people.

Rheumatoid Arthritis: The Basics

for ten years. These kinds of statistics prompt many patients to ask, "Isn't rheumatoid arthritis the 'crippling arthritis'?"

Fortunately, the news is not so bad these days. If RA is diagnosed and treated promptly there is no reason why patients should become "crippled" or disabled. The large majority of patients who are unable to work become disabled during their first few years of the disease. This fact merely emphasizes the importance of seeking early treatment during this window of opportunity to control the disease process. Early treatment can prevent permanent joint damage and muscle weakness. By contrast, a lack of adequate treatment or noncompliance with treatment (that is, not taking your medications as prescribed) are leading factors contributing to disability.

Early treatment of RA can prevent permanent joint damage and muscle weakness.

Obviously, a person with RA may find it more difficult to continue to perform a physically demanding job, such as factory work, than to stay with a more sedentary job. If you think you won't be able to continue to work at your current job, it might be a good idea to take stock of the other sorts of job skills you have or to consider retraining. Government vocational rehabilitation training programs can be a good resource for you. Obtaining Social Security disability benefits is a very slow and frustrating process and should be considered a last resort.

I became disabled and unable to work at age 58. I do agree with your risk factors in this question. But in my own case not taking medications as prescribed was not a factor. Not taking meds as prescribed is a fool's errand.

—Jim

8. Is rheumatoid arthritis a genetic disease?

Rheumatoid arthritis is affected by genes, but this disease is not controlled by a single gene. As a result, RA generally does not run in families. Instead, scientists believe that RA develops as a result of a complex interaction of genetic and environmental factors. Each person is born with a unique genetic code and has unique environmental exposures. Therefore, even if one of your family members has this disease, your own chances of developing RA are still quite low.

Examining studies of RA development in twins may help to illustrate this point. In some studies of twins, concordance was found—that is, both twins developed RA. If the twins were identical and one twin developed RA, then the chance that the other twin would develop RA was 30%. If the twins were fraternal (not identical) and one of them developed RA, then the chance that the other twin would develop RA was only 5%. From these studies, we can see that while genes have some influence on the chance of developing RA, the risk is still small.

Human leukocyte **antigens** (HLAs) are proteins on the surface of white blood cells that are associated with the body's immune system. These markers serve as a sort of genetic fingerprint, helping the body recognize infections or tissue transplants that are considered "foreign." Some HLA markers, such as HLA-DR4, are associated with more severe RA or with complications of RA such as **vasculitis** (an inflammation of the blood vessels).

Antigen

A foreign protein or carbohydrate complex that causes an immune response.

Vasculitis

Inflammation of blood vessels.

Because many people with RA don't have these markers in their blood, and because many people without RA do have these markers in their blood, HLA-based tests do not provide conclusive proof that someone has RA. Therefore doctors don't typically order this type of test; rather, the tests are generally used for research purposes. HLA-DR4 is one of the best-known genetic associations with RA, but other, less common associations have been identified as well.

Many people know that their parents had arthritis, but a reliable diagnosis of the parent's condition is not available. Your chances of "inheriting" RA from your parents are small, but if you have questions, consult your doctor.

Rheumatoid Arthritis: The Basics

I have a fraternal twin brother who had the same RA and was on the identical medication. He didn't follow the doctor's advice and died of a massive heart attack in 1999. (This was a man on a fool's errand.)

—Jim

9. Is rheumatoid arthritis caused by cigarette smoking?

The results of several large studies conducted in the past two decades support the association between cigarette smoking and the development of RA.

In one study, researchers in Finland studied 512 patients with RA. They found that men who smoked in the past but had stopped smoking were 2½ times more likely to develop RA than those who never smoked. For men who were currently smoking, the risk of RA was almost 4 times greater.

In Manchester, England, medical scientists evaluated the risk of smoking in pairs of twins where one twin had RA and the other did not. These scientists used a questionnaire to record information about the twin's smoking history. They found that if one of the pair of twins smoked, the other was also likely to smoke. In those twin pairs where one twin smoked and the other didn't, the smoker had a much higher risk of developing RA than the twin who didn't smoke. This was true in both identical twin and fraternal twin pairs.

In the United States, doctors studied the medical records of more than 30,000 women between the ages of 55 and 69 years who had enrolled in the Iowa Women's Health Study. These physicians found that the incidence of RA was almost double in those women who were currently smokers as compared to the incidence in nonsmokers. The risk of developing RA also appeared to be lower for former smokers as compared to current smokers; the risk of RA was higher in the former smokers as compared to those who never smoked. For women who had stopped smoking at least ten years prior to the start of the study, however, this risk was decreased to the same level as the risk for women who had never smoked. The U.S. doctors were not able to give a definitive reason for the association between smoking and RA in women. Some investigators in this study suggested that an interaction between the inhaled smoke and the woman's immune system might be the culprit. Others suggested that smoking might lower the level of estrogen, which in turn might increase the risk of RA. These researchers also mentioned that in other related studies, smoking was shown to raise the level of rheumatoid factor in the body.

These studies indicate that cigarette smoking significantly increases the risk of RA in both men and women. This risk of developing RA can be added to the long list of problems associated with tobacco use, such as lung, mouth, and throat cancer; emphysema; and heart disease. If you use tobacco, please discuss options for quitting with your physician. Quitting can save your joints and your life.

10. Can gum disease cause rheumatoid arthritis?

In the early part of the twentieth century, many people believed that RA was caused by dental infections. Infections of the teeth and gums were thought to spread to the joints, causing inflammation and other symptoms of RA. For example, researchers made correlations between increases in the rate of diagnosis of RA and increases in sugar consumption (a factor in periodontal disease) in England and the United States between the years 1765 and 1859.

This belief was so common that, when a patient was diagnosed with RA during this era, dentists were often employed to find and treat the dental infections that supposedly were causing it. Often, all of a patient's teeth would be removed

Rheumatoid Arthritis: The Basics

in an effort to eradicate the infection and "cure" the arthritis. While this procedure wasn't effective in curing RA, belief in the infectious theory of RA persisted. Over time, interest in this theory eventually waned as studies revealed that RA was controlled by the body's immune system. Therapy was then directed at controlling the inflammation rather than looking for dental infections.

Studies of large populations still show an association between RA and diseases of the teeth and gums, however. Medical researchers, however, have proposed alternative theories about the source of this observed association of RA and diseases of the teeth and gums. Perhaps gum disease and RA occur together because RA makes using a toothbrush difficult. Tooth and gum disease might result from being unable to effectively brush and floss one's teeth. Furthermore, patients who have RA take many medications that can affect the teeth.

Many studies have been undertaken to compare the rates of tooth plaque and dental caries (cavities) in two populations—one group consisting of patients with RA and the other group consisting of age- and sex-matched people without RA. While researchers found that the rates of dental caries and plaque were the same, RA patients had a higher level of periodontal disease and a higher rate of tooth loss. Based on these findings, some scientists have suggested that bacterial infections around the teeth can trigger a chain of events in genetically susceptible individuals that ultimately results in RA. The bacteria interact with proteins and white blood cells in the body, "tricking" the white blood cells into creating an inflammatory reaction with the body's **connective tissue.**

Connective tissue

The material that holds various body structures together. Cartilage, tendons, ligaments, and blood vessels are composed entirely of connective tissue.

While some intriguing evidence supports this theory, the jury is still out on whether it is a significant cause of RA.

PART TWO

Your Rheumatoid Arthritis Treatment Team

Which type of doctor should I see
for my rheumatoid arthritis?

Is there a difference between a medical
internist and a rheumatologist?

Do I need to see a specialist to get the best
care for my rheumatoid arthritis?

More . . .

11. Which type of doctor should I see for my rheumatoid arthritis?

Most people with RA are treated by either an internist or a rheumatologist.

Most people with RA are treated by either an internist or a rheumatologist. Who you choose to be your treating physician depends on many factors:

- The doctor's training and experience
- His or her board certification
- The proximity of the physician's office to your home
- Whether the physician participates in your insurance plan
- The doctor's reputation in the community
- Your ability to build a trusting relationship with the physician
- The doctor's ability to speak your native language or understand your culture and customs

While many of these issues do not necessarily bear directly on a doctor's knowledge or clinical abilities, patients often choose a doctor based on what is most important to them. The issue of which type of doctor a patient with RA should see for treatment has been examined in the medical literature, and differences in care and in the outcomes of patients have been noted.

Tumor necrosis factor (TNF)

A protein that plays an early and major role in the rheumatic disease process.

In studies of RA treatment practices, as compared to the care rendered by internists, rheumatologists treated patients more frequently with intensive therapies, including disease-modifying antirheumatic drugs, immunomodulators, and **tumor necrosis factor (TNF)** inhibitors (Part 5 of this book discusses the medications prescribed for RA in more detail). Furthermore, patients who were treated by rheumatologists were more likely to be referred to specialists such as rehabilitation doctors and orthopedic surgeons. As a result, these patients received more joint injections and joint replacements than their counterparts who were treated by internists and general practitioners. Overall, being treated by a rheumatologist was associated with less RA-related disability. One medical study showed that the tendency to become disabled over time was also higher among patients who made fewer than 7 visits per year to their physician than among patients who made 7 to 11 visits annually. This finding suggests that patients might have had less disability if they had visited their rheumatologist more frequently.

The more intensive level of care rendered by rheumatologists may result in improved symptoms and fewer visits to the hospital for patients with RA. Not surprisingly, however, this more intensive management leads to significantly higher costs than the costs for patients who are treated by internists.

I have always been under the care of a rheumatologist and advise anyone with RA to do the same for many reasons. When I was going through my bypass problems I was surprised to learn that the surgeons did not know the makeup of my RA meds. They had to contact my RA doctor for clarification. Rheumatologists are more aware and understand your symptoms thus provide a higher quality of care. Let's face it, that's their specialty.

—Jim

12. Is there a difference between a medical internist and a rheumatologist?

It may be helpful to understand what it means to be an internist and a rheumatologist before you choose a physician to help you with your RA.

An internist is a person who has completed four years of college, four years of medical school, and at least three years of a medical residency. During that residency, the internist studies the diagnosis and medical treatment of a wide variety of diseases affecting the human body, with emphasis on the heart, lungs, digestive track, neurological system (brain and nerves), and endocrine system (which includes the thyroid, pancreas,

Your Rheumatoid Arthritis Treatment Team

and pituitary glands). During the residency, the physician's performance is assessed by the residency training director through oral and written examinations and direct observation of the resident during his or her patient care activities.

After completing the residency, the physician is invited by the American Board of Internal Medicine to take an examination that will demonstrate his or her understanding of the skills and knowledge required to practice internal medicine. This board certification exam is a grueling two-day experience. The successful completion of this examination entitles the physician to be called "board certified" or "a diplomate of the American Board of Internal Medicine."

The American Board of Internal Medicine created this certification process to assure the public that a physician is competent to provide a high quality of patient care. Certification requirements include the following:

- Completion of a course of study leading to the M.D. or D.O. (Doctor of Osteopathy) degree from a recognized school of medicine or school of osteopathy
- Completion of a minimum of three years of required training in an accredited internal medicine residency program
- Documentation of the individual's successful performance during the residence program
- An unrestricted license to practice medicine
- Passing the American Board of Internal Medicine's certification examination

A board-certified internist is capable of rendering excellent care to patients with RA.

The rheumatologist's role is primarily to diagnose and treat individuals with arthritis and musculoskeletal diseases. These diseases include the many forms of arthritis, diffuse connective tissue diseases, autoimmune and immunologic disorders, metabolic bone diseases, and diffuse or localized musculo-skeletal pain problems. These diseases are often complex, involve multiple organ systems, and are difficult to diagnose. Their treatments can be complicated and may entail specific requirements for monitoring therapy to assure its effectiveness and avoid unwanted **side effects**.

An internist can become a rheumatologist by undertaking a **rheumatology** fellowship—an extra two to three years of medical training that focuses on the immune system and diseases of the muscles, bones, and joints. The rheumatologist spends years of in-depth study learning about arthritis and related diseases. After successfully completing the fellowship, the rheumatologist is invited to sit for a full-day examination by the American Board of Internal Medicine in rheumatological diseases. If the physician passes the test, he or she is referred to as being a "board-certified rheumatologist" or "diplomate of the American Board of Internal Medicine, Rheumatology." As a general rule, the rheumatologist will have more training and experience in the area of RA than an internist will.

13. Do I need to see a specialist to get the best care for my rheumatoid arthritis?

Most people with RA are treated by either a medical internist or a rheumatologist. Which one a patient chooses as his or her treating physician depends on many factors:

- The physician's training and experience in caring for patients with RA
- His or her board certification
- The proximity of the physician's office to your home
- Whether the physician participates in your insurance plan
- The doctor's reputation in the community
- Your ability to build a trusting relationship with the physician

Side effects
A term associated with medical treatments; problems that occur when a treatment has consequences that go beyond the desired effect, or when the patient develops problems that occur in addition to the desired therapeutic effect.

Rheumatology
The branch of medicine devoted to the study and treatment of connective tissue diseases.

Your Rheumatoid Arthritis Treatment Team

- The doctor's ability to speak your native language or understand your culture and customs

While many of these issues do not necessarily bear directly on a doctor's clinical abilities, patients will often choose a doctor based on what is most important to them. Medical internists are specialists. They have training and experience in caring for common **rheumatic diseases** such as RA, and they are qualified to provide care for typical cases of RA. Nevertheless, the amount of training and experience that an internist has is less than that of a rheumatologist.

Rheumatologists are subspecialists. Their practice is limited to people who suffer from acute and chronic musculoskeletal diseases, one of the most common of which is RA. Treating these musculoskeletal diseases often requires complicated therapeutic regimens. These regimens typically require the use of multiple medications, such as nonsteroidal anti-inflammatory medications, corticosteroids, **immunosuppressive therapy,** and the newer biological therapies. These treatments have significant risks, so their use requires close monitoring. Rheumatologists regularly collaborate with providers of physical and occupational therapy, orthopedic surgeons, and vocational rehabilitation specialists, all in an effort to make sure their patients receive the best care and have the best chance at recovery.

A consultation with a rheumatologist may be necessary in any of the following circumstances:

- After careful examination and appropriate testing, your primary care physician is unsure of the diagnosis.
- Your arthritis is unusually severe or disabling.
- Your arthritis extends beyond your joints and affects other parts of your body such as your skin, eyes, lungs, or heart.
- Your arthritis is complicated with another disease such as gout, heart disease, or kidney disease.

Rheumatic disease

Any one of more than 100 disorders that cause inflammation in connective tissues.

Immunosup-pressive therapy (immunosuppressant)

An agent capable of suppressing the immune response. Such medications increase a person's risk for infection and malignancy.

- Your RA symptoms are getting worse despite treatment.
- Your arthritis requires treatments that your primary care physician is unfamiliar with or uncomfortable administering, such as chemotherapeutic, immunosuppressive, or biological agents.

Unfortunately, many types of rheumatic diseases may not be readily identified in the early stages of the illness. Whether your condition is simple or complex, prompt diagnosis and early treatment are important both for your comfort and for your long-term well-being. In some cases, when RA is untreated or inadequately treated for a long time, injuries to the joints can occur that result in permanent disability or necessitate joint replacement.

14. My doctor suggested that I see a physical therapist. What is a physical therapist, and why do I need one?

Physical therapy is the treatment of injuries or disorders using physical methods, such as exercise, massage, or the application of heat. Ultrasound and iontophoresis (discussed later in this question) are other modalities employed by physical therapists. A physical therapist provides these treatments as well as education, instruction, and support for continued mobility.

The goal of physical therapy for people with RA is to get the individual back to the point where he or she can perform normal, everyday activities without difficulty. To reach these goals, the physical therapist may use a variety of techniques.

To Provide Pain Relief

- The application of heat packs or heated baths may be used to reduce muscle aches and improve blood circulation to the muscles and other soft tissues.

The goal of physical therapy for people with RA is to get the individual back to the point where he or she can perform normal, every-day activities without difficulty.

- The application of ice packs may be used to reduce swelling and relieve pain.
- Ultrasound is a technique that uses high-frequency sound waves to increase circulation and reduce pain. These sound waves are transferred to a specific body area via a round-headed probe. They travel deep into tissue (for example, into the muscles), creating gentle heat. In the past, a version of ultrasound termed short-wave diathermy was used as therapy for RA, but it is seldom employed today.
- Iontophoresis is the process by which drugs—usually dexamethasone and lidocaine—are propelled through the skin into a joint or small body part using a low-level electrical current. This process is noninvasive and painless, and it eliminates the potential side effects and adverse reactions that can occur with medications delivered orally or by injection.

To Preserve a Good Range of Motion

- Stretching can increase the range of motion around joints and reduce stress on the joints.
- Manual therapy, including massage, may improve or maintain the range of motion.

To Improve Strength and Cardiac Conditioning

- Aerobic exercises, including cycling and limited walking, promote good physical conditioning.
- Exercises such as lifting weights and calisthenics may strengthen muscles and improve mobility. Stronger muscles can better stabilize a weakened joint.
- Water exercises and exercising in a heated pool provide buoyancy that allows your body to exercise without placing pressure on the joints or the spine. This type of exercise is particularly helpful for people with arthritis in their lower back or legs.

To Educate

- Your physical therapist will provide you with information on which exercises are safe to perform at home and when you should not exercise, such as during periods of severe joint inflammation.
- The physical therapist can make you aware of areas in your body that need extra work to achieve or maintain mobility.

Physical therapists are professionals who have undergone special training and been certified by a state or accrediting body to design and implement physical therapy programs. They usually obtain a college education and then enter a master's degree program in physical therapy, which can last two to three years. Physical therapists work in a variety of institutions, including hospitals, clinics, and rehabilitation centers. They may also work in schools providing assistance to special education students. Finally, some work as independent practitioners who provide therapy in doctors' offices or patients' homes.

Physical therapy is often prescribed by physicians treating RA. Given that RA is a chronic disease that can result in fatigue, stiffness, and immobility, a regular program of exercise and stretching is necessary to increase joint mobility, maintain strength, and prevent weight gain. If your doctor has not suggested this type of therapy, it is a good idea to discuss this topic with him or her.

Physical Therapy—A good physical therapist can evaluate and choose the correct way to reach their goals. I find that application of heat to my sore joints is often my first self treatment. When I'm stiff and aching, I soak my hands in water that is as hot as I can stand it. I use a heating pad for my feet, shoulders, and knees. I use the type of heating pad that has a thermostat, so I can manually control the amount of heat. You should be careful not to fall asleep while using the heating pad, as it can burn your skin.

—Jim

15. What is an occupational therapist, and why does my doctor want me to see one?

People with RA may suffer significant physical, personal, familial, social, and vocational consequences from this disease. The limitations caused by RA, for example, may make performing even routine tasks more difficult. The occupational therapist's goal is to help you maintain your independence and overcome any limitations that RA has imposed on you by facilitating task performance and decreasing the consequences of RA in terms of your daily life activities. Occupational therapy is an important part of arthritis treatment plans, and the occupational therapist is an integral member of the team working to combat the effects of arthritis.

The occupational therapist's goal is to help you maintain your independence and overcome any limitations that RA has imposed on you by facilitating task performance and decreasing the consequences of RA in terms of your daily life activities.

An occupational therapist is a trained and licensed healthcare professional. To become an occupational therapist, an individual must have a college degree as well as specialized training in the form of a master's-level course in occupational therapy. Occupational therapists must pass a national examination in occupational therapy to become licensed.

Occupational therapists are usually based in hospitals or rehabilitation centers, though some make home visits. You may be evaluated by an occupational therapist after you have been given a referral from your rheumatologist.

The occupational therapist begins by taking a thorough medical and functional history. This evaluation concentrates on your ability to perform everyday life activities such as self-care, work, and leisure activities. The occupational therapist will ask specific questions about your ability to bathe, get dressed, prepare and eat meals, perform your job, play sports, or enjoy hobbies. To gain insight into your needs, he or she may also carry out a comprehensive home and job site evaluation, looking for physical challenges that those environments may pose. In addition, the therapist will conduct an extensive physical examination that concentrates on your range of motion and the observation of deformities that might hinder your performance of everyday activities.

Once the occupational therapist has assessed any limitations caused by arthritis, he or she can suggest adaptations that might make your life easier. Adaptations that the occupational therapist might suggest include the following:

- *Education and training.* You may be trained to move or do your daily chores in a way that limits joint stress and maximizes mechanical advantage. Emphasis is placed on conserving energy by balancing work and rest periods so as to optimize your efforts.
- *Splints.* The occupational therapist identifies joints that would benefit from splinting. Medical studies have shown that people who wear splints have less pain than people who do not wear splints. Splints are also useful for preventing or correcting joint deformities in the fingers or other joints. The therapist can help design specific splints to help you.
- *Assistive devices.* Devices such as zipper extensions, built-up handles on tools and utensils, and raised toilet seats can make life easier for people with RA-related limitations. Your occupational therapist may be able to help you create assistive devices for your unique needs.

An occupational therapist may be instrumental in helping someone with RA maintain his or her ability to live and work independently. Discuss your need for occupational therapy with your doctor.

16. My doctor has suggested that I see a vocational counselor. Why would I need to have a vocational counselor for my rheumatoid arthritis?

RA is a serious, progressive, and sometimes debilitating disease. By the time most people with RA have been correctly diagnosed, they have already experienced some joint damage and decreased physical ability. In some cases, these individuals' jobs may expose them to increased joint stress or they may no longer be able to perform their work owing to RA-related pain, fatigue, or loss of motion in a joint. With these issues in mind, your physician may recommend that you see a vocational counselor.

A vocational counselor is a professional with a college degree and frequently a master's degree. Such a person has received specific training in vocational counseling; in many states, he or she must also be certified. These healthcare professionals are responsible for counseling clients and maintaining professional contacts with voluntary, community, public, and private agencies for the purpose of identifying employment possibilities and engaging in job development and placement. To do so, vocational counselors work closely with local businesses and industries to elicit their cooperation for the placement of the counselors' clients in the workforce.

The vocational counselor tries to make sure that there is an adequate fit between you and your work. To determine whether this fit is right, the counselor will seek information on the following topics: your current abilities, any current difficulties that you have in performing your duties at work that are the result of your RA, your education and job training history, your personal interests and motivation, and your financial needs.

To further investigate the fit between you and your job, the vocational counselor will work cooperatively with you, your doctor, and your employer. Other assistance provided by the counselor may include testing your interest and aptitude for various jobs, a process called occupational exploration.

After a thorough evaluation, the vocational counselor should provide you with a realistic appraisal of your abilities and potential. Based on this appraisal, you can seek a job that will enable you to become employable and self-sustaining. The vocational counselor may want to speak with your current employer to see whether your old job can be temporarily or permanently changed to meet your needs. If not, the counselor can investigate other job options with your employer. Failing that, the vocational counselor will assess your skills in preparation for a new job. The counselor may suggest new employment goals based on your projected abilities or recommend educational or training facilities to help you change career paths. Through this journey, the vocational counselor remains in contact with you, monitors your career progress after job placement, and determines whether further training or job modification is appropriate.

Your Rheumatoid Arthritis Treatment Team

PART THREE

Rheumatoid Arthritis: Not Just a Disease of the Joints

My rheumatoid arthritis makes me
very tired. Is that normal?

Can rheumatoid arthritis affect my lungs?

Can rheumatoid arthritis affect my brain?

More . . .

17. My rheumatoid arthritis makes me very tired. Is that normal?

Fatigue

A condition characterized by a lessened capacity for work and reduced efficiency of accomplishment, usually accompanied by a feeling of weariness and tiredness.

Fatigue is characterized by a lack of energy and motivation. While this symptom is not as commonly discussed as the pain and stiffness associated with RA, it can be just as devastating.

Fatigue is a common feature of RA and occurs in most patients. As individuals with RA know all too well, fatigue is different from drowsiness. Fatigue is a feeling of weariness, tiredness, or lack of energy, whereas drowsiness is a lack of alertness and a feeling that you need to sleep. In other words, fatigue is characterized by a lack of energy and motivation. While this symptom is not as commonly discussed as the pain and stiffness associated with RA, fatigue can be just as devastating. For example, some patients complain of severe fatigue four to six hours after waking. This problem keeps them from being able to hold a job or even accomplish things at home.

The fatigue of RA is different from the fatigue most people feel after performing strenuous work or not getting enough sleep. The fatigue associated with RA often occurs despite adequate sleep and nutrition and lasts much longer than typical fatigue. This symptom has many causes, and a patient may suffer from more than one of these causes at the same time:

- *The inflammatory process itself.* The body of a person with RA is busy making extra white blood cells and extra inflammatory chemicals that result in the pain and swelling of joints associated with RA. The energy expended while making these mediators saps the energy that might be otherwise spent getting dressed in the morning or walking the dog.
- *Chronic pain.* Chronic joint pain means that a person walks, lifts, carries, and accomplishes other physical tasks less efficiently. It takes more energy to do less work when you have RA.
- *Poor sleep quality.* The pain and stiffness of RA result in a shorter duration of sleep and more frequent awakenings during the night.
- *Depression.* RA changes a person's life. These changes can have negative repercussions on employment, rela-

tionships, and feelings of self-esteem. As a result, the patient may experience feelings of hopelessness and helplessness and a lack of motivation.

- *Anemia.* Patients with RA can develop low red blood cell counts. This condition, which is called the "anemia of chronic disease," results from the inflammatory process that causes RA. Additionally, some of the medications that are commonly prescribed for RA can result in low blood counts owing to their effects on the bone marrow; others may cause stomach ulcers and bleeding.
- *Lack of exercise.* The pain and stiffness of RA keep many patients from participating in exercise programs or even taking a walk. Lack of exercise leads to muscle weakness, which in turn causes the individual to expend more energy doing a task than when he or she was exercising regularly and was in better shape.

Fatigue is very common in patients with RA and can be disabling. Nevertheless, this symptom is treatable in most cases. You should discuss the amount of fatigue you have with your physician. Your doctor can offer advice on how to deal with or eliminate the fatigue. It is especially important to notify your physician of any sudden worsening in your level of fatigue, as such a change may signal a disease flare, depression, or a drug side effect.

I was fortunate in my final working days to have the type of job where I could take power naps for about 1/2 to 3/4 hour when I felt the need. It was a big help and a relief from stress. People with RA learn to adapt to their disabilities and weaknesses and work around them.

—Jim

18. Can rheumatoid arthritis affect my lungs?

RA can affect the lungs and the lining of the lungs, a complication referred to as rheumatoid lung disease. Rheumatoid lung disease occurs in approximately 25% of all patients with RA.

Rheumatoid lung disease occurs in approximately 25% of all patients with RA.

Although RA occurs more commonly in women, men with RA seem to get rheumatoid lung disease more frequently. Other risk factors for this problem include smoking and development of severe joint symptoms early in the course of the disease.

Rheumatoid lung disease is not a single disease, but rather a collection of diseases of the lung that are caused by RA. The most common rheumatoid lung diseases are interstitial lung disease and pleural effusions.

Interstitial lung disease affects the lung tissue itself. In this disease, the air sacs (alveoli) of the lungs and their supporting structures become scarred by inflammation. As a consequence of the scarring, the lungs work less efficiently and it becomes harder to breathe.

Pleural effusions comprise a collection of fluid around the lung. In this condition, the lining of the lung, called the pleura, becomes inflamed and produces fluid. This is similar to the way the joints of a person with RA become inflamed and swollen with fluid. If a large amount of fluid collects around the lung, it can compress the lung and make it difficult to breathe.

The symptoms of rheumatoid lung disease include shortness of breath, cough (usually without producing sputum or phlegm), chest pain (which is worse when taking deep breaths), and fever. Your physician may also hear "crackling" sounds or a "rubbing" when he or she listens to your lungs with a stethoscope. These are not universal findings in all patients with RA, however. Decreased breath sounds or normal breath sounds can occur, even with severe lung disease.

If your physician suspects that you may have rheumatoid lung disease, he or she may order the following tests:

- *Pulmonary function test.* This test measures how much air your lungs can hold and how fast your lungs can expel the air.

- *X-rays.* A chest x-ray or a computerized tomography (CT) scan may show abnormalities consistent with rheumatoid lung disease.
- *Echocardiogram.* An echocardiogram examines your heart using sound waves. It may show that the heart is having difficulty pushing blood through the scarred lungs, a condition called pulmonary hypertension.
- *Thoracentesis of pleural effusions.* A needle is inserted into fluid around the lung and a sample is taken. Examination of this fluid may show characteristics of rheumatoid lung disease.
- *Lung biopsy.* A lung biopsy may show findings consistent with rheumatoid lung disease. The biopsy can be performed by inserting a needle through the chest wall, threading a flexible scope through the mouth and into the lungs, or conducting chest surgery to obtain an "open lung" biopsy.

The cause of rheumatoid lung disease is not well understood, though it is believed to be related to the generalized inflammatory process that occurs in the joints of a person with RA. Methotrexate (a medication that is often prescribed to treat RA) has been associated with lung fibrosis on rare occasions. Shortness of breath or chest pain in patients who are taking methotrexate as RA therapy should prompt a physician's evaluation.

Currently, there are no effective treatments for rheumatoid lung disease. Physicians sometimes prescribe corticosteroids and immunosuppressive therapies to help treat the complications of this disease.

Worsening of lung fibrosis has been described in patients who were taking antitumor necrosis factor (TNF) inhibitors, such as Humira, Enbrel, and Remicade. Although we do not know if these agents cause a worsening of the lung disease, physicians should discuss this risk with their patients who

Rheumatoid Arthritis: Not Just a Disease of the Joints

have signs of rheumatic lung disease and who are considering treatment with these agents.

19. Can rheumatoid arthritis affect my brain?

An exceedingly rare complication of prolonged, untreated RA is an inflammation of the arteries in the brain. People who experience this problem can present with symptoms similar to a stroke, such as weakness or numbness of their arms or legs. This condition can be treated with medications such as corticosteroids.

Fatigue, malaise, and depression are also commonly associated with RA. Effective treatment of RA frequently helps people feel as if they have more of their normal energy. Antidepressants may be necessary to treat depression, or they may be prescribed to help manage chronic pain.

Many of the medications used to treat arthritis have central nervous system (CNS) side effects. Corticosteroids (such as prednisone and Medrol) frequently cause nervousness, mood disturbances, and insomnia. Psychosis can also occur, although this severe side effect is usually seen only with doses of corticosteroids that are higher than those typically prescribed for RA.

Nonsteroidal anti-inflammatory drugs (NSAIDs)
Medications that relieve joint pain and stiffness by reducing inflammation. Examples include aspirin and ibuprofen.

Nonsteroidal anti-inflammatory drugs (NSAIDs) may also cause CNS side effects, albeit more subtle symptoms than those mentioned previously. Headache may be a CNS-related side effect of NSAIDs, for example. This outcome is somewhat ironic, because many of these medications are touted as headache remedies! Difficulty concentrating can also be a side effect of NSAIDs, but is often missed if the doctor and patient aren't on the lookout for it. These side effects may be more common in older people as well as with older drugs such as indomethacin.

Aspirin and other salicylates (such as salsalate and choline magnesium trisalicylate) frequently cause problems with tinnitus. Tinnitus is usually described as "ringing in the ears," but some people have much more colorful auditory experiences. For example, some people may find that tinnitus is like the sensation that there is a radio playing in the next room, for example, or it may sound like people are talking somewhere in a low murmur. Salicylates do not cause visual hallucinations, but difficulty hearing and occasionally dizziness can occur with these medications. Many older people already have some degree of tinnitus and hearing loss and aren't bothered by these medications. In other patients, the problems are additive such that a person who was mildly hard of hearing can return to the doctor's office quite deaf after taking salicylates! The doctor may monitor your blood salicylate levels if he or she suspects this kind of problem, but often it is faster and easier to just decrease the medication dosage or stop the medication temporarily. Once the salicylate level drops, the side effects of tinnitus, hearing loss, or dizziness should resolve promptly.

If you think you are having one of these side effects, speak to your doctor or pharmacist. Changing to a different medication or reducing the dose can often make a big difference.

20. Are dry eyes and dry mouth common in rheumatoid arthritis?

Some patients with RA may develop dry eyes and a dry mouth, but these are not unusual symptoms linked only with this disease. Indeed, nearly one third of all elderly people— with or without RA—will report dry eyes and dry mouth to their physician. Symptoms of dryness can result from the aging process or from taking common medications, such as antidepressants, beta blockers, diuretics, and antihistamines. Alternatively, these symptoms may be the manifestation of a disease that occurs in approximately 10% to 15% of patients with RA, called Sjögren's syndrome (SS). This syndrome is named after the Swedish eye doctor who first described it, Dr. Henrik Sjögren's (pronounced "show-grin").

Autoimmune disorder

A disorder that results when the body's tissues are attacked by its own immune system. Rheumatoid arthritis and systemic lupus erythematosus are examples of autoimmune disorders.

Like RA, SS is a chronic **autoimmune disorder.** Indeed, it is one of the most prevalent autoimmune disorders, affecting as many as 4 million Americans. It strikes both men and women, but affects women in disproportionate numbers: Approximately 90% of all people with SS are female. The men who develop this disorder typically have milder disease. The syndrome usually develops between a person's thirties and forties, but has been reported in all age groups. Approximately 50% of patients with SS have RA or another rheumatological condition, such as lupus or systemic sclerosis. In people with RA, the symptoms of SS tend to develop five to ten years after the arthritic symptoms. The cause of SS is unknown.

Whereas a person's immune cells attack the joints in RA, the immune cells attack and destroy the glands that produce tears and saliva in SS. As a result, the hallmark symptoms of this syndrome are dry mouth and dry eyes. These symptoms tend to become worse with age.

Patients with SS complain of dry eyes that may become red, itchy, and painful. The most common complaint is a gritty or sandy sensation in the eyes. These symptoms tend to worsen throughout the day. The eyelids may become inflamed. In the morning, the eyelashes can become matted (stuck together), making it difficult to open the eyes.

In addition, SS affects the mouth. Patients may complain of their tongue sticking to the roof of their mouth or an inability to eat dry food, such as crackers. Speaking may also be more difficult because of dryness. Affected individuals may mention that they need to keep a glass of water by their bedside because they frequently wake up with a dry mouth. In women with SS, vaginal dryness may lead to pain during sexual intercourse.

Sjögren's syndrome may affect other organs including the kidneys, gastrointestinal tract, blood vessels, lungs, liver, pancreas, and central nervous system. Once damaged, these organs may generate their own symptoms.

21. Is depression a problem with rheumatic arthritis?

Depression occurs frequently in the general population and even more frequently in individuals with chronic diseases such as RA. The pain and disability associated with RA has a detrimental effect on the person's lifestyle and ability to cope with daily life. RA is frequently associated with depression or anxiety; in fact, depression occurs in 20% to 25% of all patients with RA.

Depression is a disorder that is easily missed by physicians because of its nonspecific symptoms. Thus it should be brought to the physician's attention by either the patient or his or her family or friends. Common symptoms of depression include the following:

- Changes in appetite
- Sudden loss (or gain) in weight
- Changes in sleep patterns (either sleeplessness or waking too early)
- Feelings of guilt, hopelessness, and despair
- Mental and physical fatigue
- Inability to make decisions
- Withdrawal from others
- Lack of pleasure in once-pleasurable activities
- Thoughts of death and suicide (These thoughts occur in 10% of all patients with RA.)

If depression is identified, it can be treated and the quality of the patient's life improved. Treatment of depression is the same for the people with and without RA. Treatment strategies include counseling, education, frequent patient monitoring, and medications. These therapies have a high success rate.

Depression occurs frequently in the general population and even more frequently in individuals with chronic diseases such as RA. If depression is identified, it can be treated and the quality of the patient's life improved.

Regular exercise also has a modest antidepressant effect and can be a very useful adjuvant treatment for depression.

Antidepressant medication can be a particularly useful therapeutic choice. Choosing the right antidepressant is important, and the decision should be based on your specific symptoms and tolerance for side effects. All antidepressants should elevate mood, albeit not to the same extent in all patients. If you do not obtain any relief after four to six weeks of taking a particular medication, ask your doctor to change to another option. Some antidepressants can improve chronic pain by influencing the perception of pain. Other antidepressants have a side effect of drowsiness, which can help with insomnia.

22. I have a bump on my elbow that my doctor says is a rheumatoid nodule. What is a rheumatoid nodule?

A rheumatoid nodule is a bump in the skin that is found in approximately 25% of people with RA. In fact, identifying a rheumatoid nodule in a person who has recently developed arthritis can help a doctor to make the diagnosis of RA.

These bumps are found below the surface of the skin and can be moved with your fingers in most cases. Rheumatoid nodules can be as small as a pea or as large as a golf ball. The size of the nodules can change during the course of the disease, getting larger as the activity of RA increases but then regressing when the disease is quiescent. They tend to be firm, but are not rock hard and are usually not tender to the touch. These nodules are found at pressure points on the body such as the elbows and heels as well as points where the skin is irritated or traumatized, such as the knuckles of the hands and fingers and along the back of the forearm.

The exact cause of rheumatoid nodules is unknown. Some experts have theorized that they occur as a result of a minor injury to the blood vessels in the skin. This injury triggers an abnormal immune response, which in turn causes inflammation and swelling.

Despite their name, rheumatoid nodules are not found exclusively in individuals with RA. Identical nodules are sometimes seen in patients with systemic lupus erythematosus (SLE), rheumatic fever, and other diseases. They can even be caused by the presence of foreign bodies in the skin, such as splinters.

Most patients with RA don't get rheumatoid nodules; those patients who do develop these nodules tend to have more serious RA. The nodules tend to occur after the disease has been present for several years and are usually found in patients who have a strongly positive rheumatoid factor test (see Question 47) and those with more active disease.

Patients who are treated with the medication methotrexate have noted that their nodules increase in number and appear on the fingers. These new nodules can be painful and limit hand function. Antitumor necrosis factor medications such as infliximab (brand name: Remicade) can also cause nodules to decrease in size and number, though not always.

Rheumatoid nodules are clinical predictors of joint erosion and extra-articular (non-joint-related) complications of RA involving the lungs or eyes. An inflammation of the blood vessels known as rheumatoid vasculitis can occur in patients with these nodules, for example. The presence of rheumatoid nodules often suggests a need for more aggressive treatment of the underlying RA to prevent complications. Some physicians have noted that fewer patients are developing rheumatoid nodules these days thanks to the modern aggressive treatment approaches used in RA.

For the most part, rheumatoid nodules are painless and cause few problems. Nevertheless, larger nodules can cause some problems:

Rheumatoid Arthritis: Not Just a Disease of the Joints

- Pain—if they are irritated by rubbing against clothes, shoes, or jewelry, or if they become infected
- Limited joint mobility—if they are large or too close to the joint or tendon
- Neuropathy—if they press on nearby nerves
- Ulceration—if the skin overlying the nodules breaks down, causing bleeding and pain and opening up a portal for bacteria to enter and cause an infection

When ulcerations become large, deep, and long-lasting, they can result in the formation of a fistula. A fistula is an abnormal passage between the skin's surface and the inside of a joint.

Most doctors caution patients to leave rheumatic nodules alone, unless they are painful, become infected, limit the motion of a joint, or are cosmetically unacceptable. Nodules can be removed surgically, but they tend to reoccur in as little as a few months when they are present over an area of repeated trauma. Most dermatologists recommend treating nodules by injecting them with steroids. This treatment has the advantages of being able to reduce the size of the nodule while avoiding surgery and subsequent scarring. Rheumatoid nodules occasionally resolve without medical or surgical intervention.

I have rheumatoid nodules in my elbows and knuckles. The nodules have increased. Hands are stiff and painful in the morning. Soaking in hot water or using a heating pad relieves stiffness and pain.

—Jim

23. Will my rheumatoid arthritis affect my eyes?

Most people with RA do not develop eye problems because of their RA, although approximately 25% of patients with RA will complain of some eye symptoms. The majority of these eye complaints is mild and requires only symptomatic treatment. A very small number of patients develop severe eye inflammation that can affect their vision. These problems require the attention of an eye doctor.

The most common ocular (eye-related) complaint in patients with RA is "dry eyes," also referred to by the unwieldy medical name keratoconjunctivitis sicca. This condition occurs in as many as 15% of patients and is explained in some depth in Question 20.

A less common, but more serious eye complaint is scleritis. Scleritis is a chronic, painful, and potentially blinding inflammatory disease. Its exact incidence is uncertain, though it is thought to be rare. Some studies indicate that this condition occurs in fewer than 10% of patients with RA and is usually associated with very severe cases of RA. It occurs slightly more frequently in women than men and first occurs in patients who are in their fifties or sixties.

Scleritis is characterized by swelling and redness of the white portion of the eye called the scleral and episcleral tissues. It is sometimes confused with a minor bacterial infection of the eye called "pink eye" (more formally, **conjunctivitis**) because of the bright red appearance of the eye. Your doctor can tell the difference by taking a thorough history and performing a physical examination.

Conjunctivitis
An inflammation of the outer membrane of the eye.

The most common symptoms of scleritis include pain, tearing, photophobia (pain when the eyes are exposed to bright light), and tenderness when the eye is pressed, and decreased visual acuity. The pain can be severe, so it is often the symptom that prompts someone to seek medical assistance for scleritis. The pain results from stretching of the nerve endings caused by the inflammation.

The initial treatment of scleritis focuses on relieving the eye discomfort and stopping the progression of the disease. This

Rheumatoid Arthritis: Not Just a Disease of the Joints

therapy includes common pain relievers that are taken orally (by mouth) such as indomethacin (Indocin) or ibuprofen (Motrin). If a patient doesn't respond to this treatment, he or she should be referred to an ophthalmologist (eye doctor) for stronger medical therapy. This therapy may include steroid eye drops, immunosuppressive medication such as cyclosporine, or an anti-TNF medication such as infliximab (Remicade). If scleritis is not treated, it can result in loss of vision or even the loss of the eye itself, though this occurs only in the most serious and destructive type of scleritis (called necrotizing scleritis).

Other, less common eye-related complications of RA include inflammation of the blood vessels in the eye (choroiditis), retinal detachments, and swelling of the retina (macular edema). All of these complications can result in loss of vision. For this reason, patients with RA should have regular eye exams and speak to their doctor if they experience eye redness, pain, or a change in the acuity of their vision.

24. Can rheumatoid arthritis increase my risk of osteoporosis and bone fractures?

Yes, RA can increase your risk of developing osteoporosis and bone fractures. Osteoporosis is a disease of the bones that results in "thinner," weaker bones that are more prone to fractures. It is a silent disease, however: A person can't feel that his or her bones are getting less dense. Osteoporosis becomes obvious only when the individual suffers a fracture of the hip, wrist, or spine. Osteoporosis-related fractures of the spine, for example, can result in a curvature of the spine called kyphosis ("dowager's hump"). These fractures may or may not be painful, can be disfiguring, and may result in disability and hospitalizations.

Risk factors for developing osteoporosis include the following:

• Family history of the disease
• Thinness or small frame

- Low dietary calcium intake
- Inactivity or lack of exercise
- Smoking
- Excessive alcohol intake
- Prolonged use corticosteroids
- Being postmenopausal and having an early onset of menopause

Medical studies have found that people with RA have an increased risk of bone loss and bone fracture as compared to people of the same sex and age who do not have RA. There are many reasons why people with RA might develop bone loss:

- The inflammation of RA not only causes bone loss at the joints and the areas surrounding the joints, but tends to accelerate bone loss throughout the entire skeleton.
- Women, who are at an increased risk for developing osteoporosis relative to men, are two to three times more likely than men to suffer from rheumatoid arthritis as well.
- Exercise and weight bearing tend to limit bone loss. The inactivity and lack of exercise caused by the pain, stiffness, and fatigue of RA tend to increase bone loss.
- Corticosteroids (also called glucocorticoids—for example, cortisone and prednisone) are often prescribed to decrease inflammation and ease pain. Unfortunately, if they are taken for long periods of time, these medications can cause significant bone loss.
- The pain, fatigue, and stiffness caused by RA can also impair a person's ability to walk and cause an unsteady gait. This may result in falls that can cause fractures.

Despite its "silent nature," osteoporosis is a disease that can be tested for and treated. As with RA, there is no cure for osteoporosis, but the disease can be managed. The management of

Medical studies have found that people with RA have an increased risk of bone loss and bone fracture as compared to people of the same sex and age who do not have RA. Although there is no cure for osteoporosis, the disease can be managed.

Rheumatoid Arthritis: Not Just a Disease of the Joints

osteoporosis is the same for people with RA as it is for those without RA.

To identify the presence of osteoporosis, your doctor can quantify your bone density. The bone densitometry exam or bone mineral density (BMD) test is painless and is typically performed in a doctor's office or the outpatient department of a hospital. It uses low doses of x-rays to examine the bones in your wrist, hip, and spine and to determine whether they are of a normal density or if they show signs of bone loss. Sometimes bone density of the heel is used as a screening test for osteoporosis.

You can reduce your risk of osteoporosis in several ways:

Vitamin D

A fat-soluble vitamin that causes the intestines to increase absorption and metabolism of the minerals calcium and phosphorus (the building blocks of bone).

- Increase the amount of calcium and **vitamin D** in your diet. Your doctor may recommend calcium and vitamin D supplements in the form of pills.
- Your doctor may wish to measure the level of vitamin D in your blood. If the test shows that this level is low, you can take a supplement to correct this deficiency.
- Increase the amount of exercise you do. Your bones become stronger when they are stimulated by exercise and weight bearing. Of course, you should consult your doctor before starting any new exercise program. Exercise can be avoided when your RA flares up.
- Avoid smoking and excessive alcohol intake.
- If your doctor determines that it is appropriate, he or she may prescribe one of several medications that are indicated for the treatment of osteoporosis. These medications can slow the rate of bone loss and help strengthen your bones.

Patients with RA should discuss their risk for osteoporosis with their primary care physician or rheumatologist. Even minor changes in lifestyle can reduce your risk for bone loss and fractures.

25. Can rheumatoid arthritis cause a low red blood cell count?

Anemia—an abnormally low number of red blood cells in your bloodstream—is a common complication of RA. Indeed, of all the problems associated with RA that are not related to joints, anemia is the most common. It is estimated to occur in 30% to 60% of all people with RA. Anemia tends to occur more frequently in those people who have the most severe disease, defined as a higher number of involved joints and higher levels of functional disability and pain.

Anemia has many different causes and is by no means unique to RA. Nevertheless, this complication can lead to worsening fatigue and shortness of breath in people with RA. Two types of anemia are primarily associated with RA: iron-deficiency anemia and the "anemia of chronic disease."

Iron-deficiency anemia is caused by a loss of blood. In people with RA, the most common reasons for blood loss are normal menstrual bleeding (in women) and bleeding in the gastro-intestinal (GI) tract. Gastrointestinal bleeding can be caused by taking nonsteroidal anti-inflammatory drugs (NSAIDs), such as ibuprofen or naproxen. The use of these medications is associated with gastric ulcers and sometime severe hemor-rhages. In one study of patients with both RA and anemia, iron-deficiency anemia accounted for 23% of all cases.

The majority of patients who have both RA and anemia have the "anemia of chronic disease." In this type of anemia, the abnormal chemicals and proteins that cause the joint inflam-mation in RA also affect the cells in the bone marrow that produce red blood cells. That is, they inhibit the production of new red blood cells, even though your body has enough iron to make the cells.

You doctor can determine whether you have anemia by ob-taining a simple blood test called a **complete blood count**

Complete blood count (CBC)

A test that gives information about the cells in a person's blood.

(CBC). Your doctor should perform this test several times each year and anytime you complain of increased shortness of breath or fatigue.

The treatment for anemia depends on its cause. For patients with iron-deficiency anemia, treatment of GI ulcers and re-placement of lost iron is often sufficient. Iron is usually re-placed by taking iron supplement pills.

The treatment for the anemia of chronic disease is more com-plicated. It begins with a more aggressive treatment of the in-flammation caused by the RA. Iron supplementation is rarely necessary, because people with this type of anemia usually have normal amounts of iron stored in their body. A newer treatment is erythropoietin, a synthetic form of the naturally occurring protein in our bodies that stimulates the production of red blood cells. Patients who are treated with erythropoietin sometimes experience rapid improvements in both their red blood cell counts and their symptoms of fatigue.

If you are experiencing increased fatigue or shortness of breath, discuss the possibility of anemia with your physician. A simple blood test could help to make the diagnosis.

26. I've heard that people with rheumatoid arthritis are prone to heart disease. Is that true?

Yes, patients with RA have an increased risk of developing atherosclerosis and cardiovascular disease. In particular, RA is associated with a 40% increased risk for myocardial infarction (heart attack) and a 60% increased risk for congestive heart failure (CHF). The heart disease associated with RA accounts for 30% to 50% of deaths in patients with RA. Death occurs at an earlier age in individuals with RA as compared with those without RA who have similar heart disease risk factors. By some estimates, patients with RA die 17 years earlier than people without RA.

Why people with RA have a higher rate of heart attacks is unknown. We do know that the changes that RA causes in a person's body can damage the lining of the arteries. This damage results in inflammation in the lining of the arteries, which in turn leads to cholesterol deposits. These cholesterol deposits (called atheroma or plaque) can block arteries and cause heart attacks. In addition, RA has been associated with other changes that can result in coronary artery blockages, including increased levels of cholesterol and fat (triglycerides) in the bloodstream and an increase in clotting factors.

The increased risk for heart disease observed in persons with RA is independent of the usual risk factors for heart disease, which include high cholesterol, high blood pressure, advanced age, diabetes, smoking, obesity, and family history of heart disease. The risk of heart disease has been correlated with the severity of the RA: The worse the RA, the greater the amount of inflammation, and the higher the risk of heart disease. Researchers have also found an association between an RA patient's **C-reactive protein (CRP)**, sedimentation rate (ESR), and risk for cardiovascular death: The higher the person's ESR, the higher the risk of cardiovascular death. Some researchers believe that decreasing the amount of inflammation a patient has can decrease his or her risk of heart disease. In medical studies, patients who used methotrexate or biologic agents (e.g., Remicade, Humira, and Enbrel) to treat their RA had a lower risk of heart disease. Conversely, the use of prednisone (a potent anti-inflammatory medication) tended to increase the risk of atherosclerosis and heart attack.

Individuals who have RA should be aware of their increased risk for heart attacks. They should discuss this risk with their physicians and develop a plan to modify those risks. While some heart disease risk factors cannot be modified (such as family history of heart disease), others can. You should work to reduce your modifiable risk factors for heart attacks—for example, stop smoking (if you currently smoke), follow a

---

C-reactive protein (CRP)

A type of protein that is made in the liver. The amount of CRP rises in the blood in conjunction with the inflammation produced by certain conditions.

Individuals who have RA should be aware of their increased risk for heart attacks and should work to reduce their modifiable risk factors for heart attacks.

---

low-fat diet, and exercise. Make these changes only after consulting with your physician.

Here are some questions to discuss with your physician:

- How do I stop smoking?
- How do I change my diet to reduce my fat and cholesterol intake and to achieve an optimal weight?
- Which exercises should I do, given the limitations imposed by my RA? How frequently and how long should I exercise? (Exercising 30 minutes three times per week is usually recommended.)
- Would I benefit from a cholesterol-lowering medication? A class of cholesterol-lowering drugs called statins should be evaluated in this regard. Not only can statins improve your lipid levels, but they also appear to have anti-inflammatory properties. Recent clinical trials suggest that statins offer a dual benefit of both protection against cardiovascular disease and prevention of RA progression.
- Should I take methotrexate to lower the amount of inflammation in my body?
- Will taking biologic agents such as Remicade, Humira, and Enbrel improve my arthritis and decrease my risk of heart disease?

Other heart complications associated with RA include inflammation of the heart's outer covering (pericardium) and the heart muscle (myocardium). When the pericardium is inflamed by RA, the condition is referred to as rheumatic pericarditis. Rarely, an inflammation of the heart muscle, called myocarditis, can develop. Both of these conditions can lead to CHF, which is characterized by shortness of breath and fluid accumulation in the lungs.

Individuals with RA should have their blood pressure, blood sugar level, and cholesterol level checked at least every year. For older patients or those with a family history of heart disease, an electrocardiogram (EKG) or a cardiac stress test may be indicated. If you have additional risk factors, your doctor may recommend a consultation with a cardiologist.

27. Can rheumatoid arthritis increase my risk for infections?

Infections are a frequent complication in people with RA. Their risk for developing lung infections or pneumonia is also increased, which constitutes a serious problem.

In medical studies, investigators have found that people with RA were nearly twice as likely as people without RA to develop infections, even after adjusting the rates for age, gender, smoking status, low white blood cell count, glucocorticoid use, and diabetes mellitus. The sites of infection with the highest risk ratios were the bones, joints, skin, and soft tissue.

Possible explanations for the increased risk of infection include RA-related immunologic abnormalities, the effects of immunosuppressant drugs, and disease-related factors such as immobility, joint surgery, rheumatoid lung disease, and Felty's syndrome. In addition, patients with RA who also have other diseases such as diabetes mellitus, chronic obstructive pulmonary disease (COPD), and renal failure may have an even higher risk of developing infections. Which of these factors are the most important contributors to the increased risk of infection associated with RA has not been established.

Recent evidence suggests that an abnormality exists in the white blood cells (the T cells) of patients with RA, even when the disease is in its earliest stages. This abnormality may impair the body's immunological response to bacteria and viruses, leaving it unable to fight off these intruders and resulting in increased infection rates.

Corticosteroids (or, more simply, steroids) are commonly used to treat rheumatic diseases. Unfortunately, their ability to control RA symptoms comes at the expense of increased immunosuppression, which increases the risk for infections. In one study involving nearly 17,000 people with RA, researchers found that more than 70% of patients were prescribed prednisone (a steroid) at least once during the course of their disease and 35% to 45% used prednisone regularly. Evidence from studies like this one has also indicated that there is a relationship between the dose of steroids and the risk of pneumonia. This association is seen even with small daily doses of steroids—less than 5 mg.

Disease-modifying antirheumatic drugs (DMARDs)

A class of medications that are used to treat arthritis and other rheumatic conditions. Examples include methotrexate, leflunomide, and sulfasalizine.

The use of **disease-modifying antirheumatic drugs (DMARDs,** such as sulfasalazine, hydroxychloroquine, and leflunomide), apart from corticosteroids, did not appear to increase infection risk, even after adjustment for demographic and disease-related variables. The effects of the dosages of methotrexate used in RA are less clear, with some studies showing a mildly increased risk of infection and others demonstrating no such increased risk.

28. Can rheumatoid arthritis increase my risk for a joint infection?

Although they are rare, joint infections do occur sometimes. It is important to know about this potential complication for two reasons. First, among all of the many types of arthritis, arthritis caused by infections results in the most rapid destruction of joints. In some cases, a joint can be totally destroyed after only a few days of untreated infection. Second, joint infections are often misdiagnosed, even by experienced doctors.

A joint infection is referred to as septic arthritis. Doctors suspect septic arthritis when they see intense inflammation of a joint along with cloudy fluid inside the joint. A diagnosis of septic arthritis usually requires special tests of joint fluid to determine whether microorganisms, such as bacteria, are present in the joint fluid. While bacteria cause the majority of infections, viruses, tuberculosis, and fungi can also cause this problem.

A joint that has been previously damaged by injury or arthritis is more likely to become infected than an undamaged joint. In the general population, joint infections occur at a rate of 10 cases in every 100,000 people. Among individuals with RA, this rate jumps to 70 cases in every 100,000 people.

Although septic arthritis can occur in any joint, the knee is the most common site of infection, accounting for approximately 50% of cases. The hip is the next most common site of infection, accounting for 20% of cases. The shoulders, elbows, ankles, and wrists account for the majority of the remaining cases.

Infectious agents can enter the joint from many sources, though the most common route of infection is via the blood. Bacteria from an infection in a distant location, such as the heart or lungs, can be carried to the joint by the bloodstream. Joints may also become infected during a surgical procedure, such as a joint replacement, **arthroscopy,** or even the injection of steroids into the joint. Fortunately, these complications, while serious, are very rare. Direct trauma to the joint, such as an open fracture, stepping on a nail, or having a bite wound to a knuckle can also lead to infection of a joint.

Arthroscopy

A diagnostic and surgical technique that uses a thin tube with a light and a tiny video camera at one end to view the inside of a joint.

In its earliest stages, septic arthritis can be difficult to diagnose. The joint may be sore and swollen. As the infection progresses, the symptoms become more severe. Typically, a person with a septic joint presents with fever and a joint that is hot, red, painful, and bulging. The joint is very painful to flex or extend and may even be too painful to touch. Given that this doesn't sound different from a worse-than-average flare of RA, you can see why your physician might have difficulty making this diagnosis. The following clues should point your doctor to a diagnosis of septic arthritis:

Rheumatoid Arthritis: Not Just a Disease of the Joints

- History of fever
- An inability to bear weight on the affected joint
- An elevation in your "sed rate" (sedimentation rate—specifically, an erythrocyte sedimentation rate higher than 40 mm/hour) or C-reactive protein (CRP)
- An elevated white blood cell count (WBC count higher than 12,000/liter)

Septic arthritis is diagnosed by placing a needle into the joint and aspirating the fluid for analysis. The joint fluid is then examined under a microscope. The presence of bacteria or other infectious organisms confirms the diagnosis.

The treatment of an infected joint starts with the administration of intravenous antibiotics. The joint itself needs to be drained of the excess fluid that contributes to joint destruction. This fluid is drained with a needle as often as is necessary—sometimes daily. Sometimes, the joint has to be opened and drained surgically.

Any severely inflamed joint should be examined by your doctor, especially if you also have a fever. Early treatment of an infected joint will prevent joint damage and hospitalization.

Untreated infections can rapidly destroy a joint and lead to more widespread infection; in turn, widespread infection can result in hospitalization and even death. Therefore, any severely inflamed joint should be examined by your doctor, especially if you also have a fever. Early treatment of an infected joint will prevent joint damage and hospitalization.

29. Do patients with rheumatoid arthritis have more dental problems than the average person?

Surveys of large groups of people show that individuals with RA have twice the rate of periodontal disease as people of the same age, sex, and socioeconomic status who do not have RA. Periodontal disease affects the tissues that surround and support the teeth. These tissues include the gums (gingiva), the bones that form the tooth sockets, and the periodontal

ligament (a thin layer of connective tissue that holds the tooth in its socket, and acts as a cushion between tooth and bone).

In studies, researchers have discovered that patients with RA tend to have more severe periodontal disease than those without RA. Of the patients with both RA and periodontal disease, 62.5% of them suffered from advanced disease and more than half had severe bone loss in the jaw. In addition, the patients with RA averaged 11.6 missing teeth compared with 6.7 missing teeth in the control group in one Australian study.

Both RA and periodontal disease are inflammatory diseases that lead to bone destruction. When researchers examined patients who had both RA and periodontal disease, they found that the rates of other inflammatory diseases, such as cardiovascular disease and diabetes mellitus, were higher in this group than in age-matched people without RA. They also noted a relationship between the severity of the periodontal disease and the risk of having RA: Patients with more advanced periodontal disease were at higher risk of having RA.

One theory suggests that the inflammation and infection associated with periodontal disease help to trigger RA. This relationship suggests that periodontal disease may be the result of the same inflammatory process that affects the joints of patients with RA. Other researchers have suggested that the effects of RA, such as swollen and painful fingers, loss of motion, fatigue, and decreased saliva production, result in poor oral hygiene that causes periodontal disease. Dentists cannot be sure which problem came first, but they do emphasize that good oral hygiene can decrease plaque and gingivitis. They encourage patients with RA to brush with an electric toothbrush, floss daily, and visit their dentist regularly for plaque removal and repair of dental caries (cavities) if present.

Rheumatoid Arthritis: Not Just a Disease of the Joints

30. Does rheumatoid arthritis increase a person's risk of getting cancer of the lymph nodes (lymphoma)?

Patients with RA appear to have a higher risk of developing cancers of the lymph nodes, known as lymphomas. In the past, studies have shown that the risk of developing lymphoma appears to be greater in patients who have more severe inflammation and in those with a longer duration of RA. The reasons for this increased risk are not clear, but the effects of arthritis drugs, viruses, or increased inflammation have been blamed. Many medical studies have attempted to quantify this risk and find its cause. A few of the seminal studies in this area are reviewed here.

Researchers in Canada evaluated the health records of 1210 patients with a diagnosis of RA to determine their risk of developing lymphoma. They found a three- to fourfold increase in the rate of lymphoma in these patients as compared to other Canadian patients without arthritis. This study was published in the *Journal of Clinical Epidemiology* in 1993.

In a 1998 study published in the *British Journal of Medicine,* Swedish researchers offered evidence from a population-based study that "immune alterations" in patients with RA appear to contribute to the development of lymphomas. In a population-based sample of 11,683 patients with RA in Sweden, these researchers identified 41 patients with lymphoma and 113 without the disease. They found that there was a strong independent association between the severity and duration of inflammatory activity and the risk of lymphoma. Because arthritis drugs such as methotrexate, azathioprine, and infliximab have been suspected to contribute to the risk of lymphoma, the researchers examined the drug treatments for all patients. They found no link between any specific drug used in RA and an increased risk of lymphoma. The Swedish investigators suggested that if inflammation contributed to the risk of developing lymphoma, then treatment of RA with anti-inflammatory medications might lower a patient's risk.

In 2004, a study published in the medical journal *Arthritis and Rheumatism* reaffirmed the connection between RA and lymphoma and cast doubt on the connection between arthritis drugs and this cancer. In this study of 18,572 patients with RA, researchers evaluated known and suspected risk factors for lymphoma, including age, sex, severity of RA, duration of RA, and any RA treatments received. In patients with RA, the overall risk of developing a lymphoma was twice the risk of people without RA. These investigators found that increasing age, male sex, and low educational achievement were associated with increased risk of lymphoma. Conversely, current or previous drug treatment had no effect on cancer risk.

Patients with RA should be aware that they have a slightly increased risk of developing lymphoma. Symptoms such as changes in weight, fevers, and swollen lymph nodes should be reported immediately to your physician. Those symptoms do not mean you have cancer of your lymph nodes; they can also be associated with a variety of other illnesses, including minor ailments such as colds or viruses. As in other serious illnesses, early detection and treatment of lymphoma results in improved outcomes.

Patients with RA have a slightly increased risk of developing lymphoma. Report symptoms such as changes in weight, fevers, and swollen lymph nodes immediately to your physician.

Rheumatoid Arthritis: Not Just a Disease of the Joints

PART FOUR

Treatment of Rheumatoid Arthritis: General Principles

Can my rheumatoid arthritis be
treated when I'm pregnant?

How will the doctor choose the
right medication for me?

My rheumatoid arthritis is not so bad now.
How long should I wait to treat it?

More . . .

31. Can my rheumatoid arthritis be treated when I'm pregnant?

Rheumatoid arthritis does not appear to have any adverse effects on pregnancy outcome. Some medications used to treat RA have not been thoroughly studied in pregnant women, however, and should be used with caution in this population. How a woman with RA is treated during her pregnancy is a complicated decision that should be made cooperatively by the patient, her obstetrician, and her rheumatologist. Treatment decisions require careful consideration of the risks and benefits to the mother and fetus.

During pregnancy, the joint symptoms of women with RA improve in approximately 75% of cases. Most women who improve experience initial relief in the first trimester, but RA almost invariably recurs within three to four months after delivery. A minority of pregnant patients have a significant worsening of their symptoms that requires changes in the dosages of their current medications or the addition of new medications.

Rheumatoid arthritis therapy during pregnancy is complicated because many of the drugs used to treat RA have not been adequately tested in medical studies of pregnant women. Therefore, they may be dangerous to the unborn child.

Disease-modifying antirheumatic drugs (DMARDs) such as methotrexate (Rheumatrex), sulfasalazine (Azulfidine), hydroxychloroquine (Plaquenil), leflunomide (Arava), cyclosporine (Sandimmune, Neoral), gold salts (Solganal), azathioprine (Imuran), and D-penicillamine (Cuprimine, Depen) should be stopped in women who are trying to conceive and in pregnant and lactating women. Some of these medications are more harmful than others during pregnancy; that is, evidence of the risks of these agents to the fetus either exists or cannot be ruled out. Methotrexate should be stopped in both men and women who are planning to conceive a baby because evidence suggests that it may cause birth defects (also called teratogenicity). Women who are planning to become pregnant should stop methotrexate for at least one complete ovulatory cycle before attempting conception. Men taking this drug should stop it six months prior to fathering a child.

Prednisone is an option for the treatment of pregnant women with RA. Although the use of this medication in pregnant women has been not investigated in controlled medical studies, no evidence exists that low-dose prednisone (less than 20 mg daily) used in the first two trimesters poses any risks to the fetus. If this medication is necessary, joint symptoms are best managed with the lowest possible dose of prednisone. Potential complications of prednisone use during pregnancy include worsening of maternal gestational diabetes, hypertension, and intrauterine growth retardation.

Similarly, nonsteroidal anti-inflammatory drugs (NSAIDs) can be used in the first two trimesters of pregnancy. They should be avoided in the third trimester because of their potential negative effects on the pregnancy:

- Effects on the baby's heart (premature closure of the ductus arteriosus)
- Prolonged labor
- Excessive bleeding after child birth (peripartum hemorrhage)

Although both NSAIDs and prednisone are excreted in breast milk, the American Academy of Pediatrics considers them safe for breastfeeding mothers. If NSAIDs are used, drugs with a short duration of action (a short "half-life") are preferable. Ideally, these drugs should be taken immediately after breastfeeding.

The safety of using tumor necrosis factor (TNF) inhibitors during pregnancy has not been well studied. While several case

Treatment of Rheumatoid Arthritis: General Principles

reports indicate that women have gone through normal pregnancies and delivered healthy children while on one of these drugs, the U.S. Food and Drug Administration (FDA) does not recommend the use of TNF inhibitors in pregnant women.

Men and women with RA who are considering conceiving a child should discuss their treatment options with their rheumatologists well in advance of the planned pregnancy. Women should include their obstetricians in these discussions and should inform them of any change in their medications during their pregnancy. Much useful information on medications and pregnancy can be found at the Organization of Teratology Information Specialists website (www.otispregnancy.org).

32. How will the doctor choose the right medication for me?

The goals of RA treatment have evolved in the last decade. In the past, the best that a patient could hope for was decreased pain and stiffness. Today, thanks to more effective drugs and earlier, more aggressive treatment of RA, expectations are much higher. Your doctor's goals for treatment are multifold:

- Alleviating joint-related symptoms (such as pain, swelling, and stiffness)
- Preserving function and maintaining the greatest possible mobility of the affected joints
- Preventing deformity and disability
- Improving quality of life
- Reducing the secondary effects of RA, such as clogging of the arteries (atherosclerosis), thinning of the bones (osteoporosis), and infections

At each meeting with your doctor, you should discuss your progress toward these goals. The results of this discussion will affect the choice of treatment for your RA.

Choosing the right RA medication for you involves many factors. Long ago, the approach to RA was based on a "treatment pyramid." Relatively weak medications, which served as the base of the pyramid, were used first. As symptoms worsened and only after considerable procrastination and delay, more effective medications (located higher up on the pyramid) might be prescribed. Such a gradual approach to the treatment of RA is now considered incorrect, and early, aggressive treatment of RA is now the norm. Experts have come to the conclusion that if they don't "hit it with their best shot" early on, the chances of long-term success in controlling the damage of RA will be greatly reduced.

For many patients, methotrexate is an excellent medication to start with, unless there is a specific reason not to use it. Methotrexate takes about a month to begin working. The process of gradually increasing the dose to achieve its maximum effectiveness might take a few more months. In a small number of patients, methotrexate can cause liver problems, so people who have a history of liver disease might not be able to take this medication. Also, because alcohol impairs liver function, people who drink alcoholic beverages regularly may not be good candidates for this medication. Methotrexate can cause birth defects or miscarriage, so it can be used only by women of childbearing potential who promise to employ reliable birth control.

For people with mild cases of RA, it is sometimes possible to prescribe medications that are "user friendly" in terms of the requirements for lab work (needed for monitoring) and follow-up office visits. Those medications might include NSAIDs, hydroxychloroquine, or sulfasalazine. There are many possible exceptions or special circumstances that might influence which particular medication is chosen for a particular person.

For many people with RA, a combination of medications is needed to control their disease. The general goal with such

Early, aggressive treatment of RA is now the norm. Experts have concluded that if they don't "hit it with their best shot" early on, the chances of long-term success in controlling the damage of RA will be greatly reduced.

Treatment of Rheumatoid Arthritis: General Principles

combination therapy is to maximize the benefits and minimize the side effects by using smaller doses of several medications instead of a larger dose of a single medication. Some combinations of medications show extra benefit when they are combined—that is, they act synergistically.

Many combinations of medications are possible, but relatively few firm guidelines have been established regarding how to combine these medications. The combination of methotrexate, hydroxychloroquine, and/or sulfasalazine is a popular choice. Azathioprine or leflunomide might also be added; because these medications and methotrexate share some side effects in common, however, there is at least a theoretical concern about additive toxicity with this regimen.

Prednisone is a powerful anti-inflammatory medication with a rapid onset. Indeed, patients often feel better after taking this steroid for just a few days. It is frequently used in combination with other RA medications. Prednisone is particularly helpful early in the treatment course, because many other RA drugs take weeks to months to reach their maximal effectiveness. Once the slower-acting medications (such as methotrexate) have had a chance to work, the prednisone dose can be gradually decreased. Because prednisone has the potential to produce numerous side effects, including weight gain, doctors usually advise, "The smallest possible dose, for the shortest duration of time." Nevertheless, this type of medication works so well that many people with RA remain on small doses of prednisone for long periods of time.

If a combination of these medications doesn't control the patient's RA symptoms or isn't tolerated because of side effects, the next step is to add one of the newer biologic medications—specifically, tumor necrosis factor (TNF) inhibitors, such as etanercept, adalimumab, or infliximab. Which biologic agent is used first depends on many factors, including your ability to inject yourself with the medication, your willingness to get an IV infusion, and your insurance company's willingness to pay for a particular medication. You should discuss the pros and cons of each medication with your doctor before beginning treatment.

These anti-TNF medications are typically used in combination with methotrexate. If one of the TNF inhibitors fails to produce acceptable results, another TNF inhibitor or one of the other biologic medications (such as kineret, abatacept, or rituximab) might be substituted into the drug regimen. Biologic medications are rarely used in combination with each other because of concerns about the increased risk of suppression of the body's immune system, which might lead to infections.

The early use of effective RA medications alone or in combination has enabled us to make great strides in our management of RA. Vast improvements have already been made, and more progress is likely in the future.

33. My rheumatoid arthritis is not so bad now. How long should I wait to treat it?

For people with RA, "watchful waiting" is not an appropriate treatment strategy. Medical studies reveal some important facts that demonstrate why early treatment of RA is necessary:

- The majority of joint destruction occurs in the first two years after disease onset.
- Significant joint destruction can occur even when the joint is not painful.
- Joint damage is irreversible—it does not "improve" significantly with treatment.
- Patients who are treated early feel better than those who delay treatment for one year.
- Patients who are treated early tend to have a more robust response to medications than those who wait for treatment.

Not all early treatments are the same, however. A Dutch study showed that the type of early treatment you receive matters. In this study, investigators compared patients with RA who were treated with therapies such as nonsteroidal anti-inflammatory drugs (NSAIDs) or methotrexate alone to other patients who were treated with combinations of methotrexate and infliximab, a tumor necrosis factor (TNF) blocker. They found that the more aggressive combination (methotrexate/infliximab) resulted in less joint erosion and improved function than in patients treated with monotherapy (a single drug). Some patients in this study actually experienced a remission of their disease; that is, after the aggressive combination treatment, they had no signs or symptoms of RA. How long these remissions will last is unknown.

While it's ideal to initiate treatment as early as possible, aggressive treatment throughout the course of the disease is essential, say experts. Even if you've passed the two-year mark and have sustained some joint damage through a lack of treatment or treatment that wasn't completely successful, you can still benefit from aggressive therapy. While some joints may have been damaged, others can be preserved by treating your RA appropriately. Further, the burden of inflammation, which results in non-joint-related RA difficulties such as an increased risk for **coronary artery disease** and stroke, can be improved by therapy. A decreased risk for these complications can be seen, even years after the start of RA symptoms.

34. I've had rheumatoid arthritis for a long time. Is it too late to treat it?

Even people with advanced RA can benefit from medical treatment. The treatment benefits can include the following:

- Reduced joint pain
- Reduced involvement of other joints

While it's ideal to initiate treatment as early as possible, aggressive treatment throughout the course of the disease is essential. Even if you've passed the two-year mark and have sustained some joint damage through a lack of treatment or treatment that wasn't completely successful, you can still benefit from aggressive therapy.

Coronary artery disease

A narrowing of the coronary arteries that results in inadequate blood flow to the heart.

- Increased mobility
- Reduced risk for cancer, heart disease, and stroke

Joint Pain

Even if a joint has undergone considerable erosion and lost some mobility, inflammation can still result in continued pain, tenderness, and disability. RA can continue to damage joints, even if they are not very painful.

Involvement of Other Joints

RA is a progressive disease. The inflammatory process may involve only a few joints today, but other joints might be involved tomorrow. Reducing the disease activity with aggressive medical treatment may prevent the involvement of other joints that could result in further pain and disability.

Mobility

Joints can be immobilized by pain, inflammation, and erosions. Current treatment can decrease this pain and inflammation of joints, which can result in an increased ability to walk, go to work, and enjoy hobbies. While current treatment may rebuild damaged joints, reducing the pain and inflammation is also worthwhile.

Systemic Risk of Heart Disease, Stroke, and Cancer

Many studies have shown that the chronic inflammation associated with RA raises a person's risk for developing heart disease, stroke, and cancer, especially cancer of the lymph nodes (lymphoma). Reducing the amount of inflammation can reduce your risk of experiencing the long-term complications of RA.

If you continue to have RA symptoms, you should discuss your treatment with your doctor. Working together, you should strive to balance the risks of continued uncontrolled inflammation against the risks of more aggressive treatment.

Treatment of Rheumatoid Arthritis: General Principles

35. Can rheumatoid arthritis be put into remission?

Remission in a person with RA can be defined as the absence of disease activity, such as swollen joints, pain, and stiffness.

In the 1980s, when the authors of this book began practicing medicine, physicians approached RA differently than they do today. Back then, physicians were mostly concerned with controlling patients' symptoms. Patients were treated with non-steroidal anti-inflammatory drugs (NSAIDs), which relieved some of their pain and were felt to be relatively safe. Physicians avoided "aggressive therapy," with its attendant risks, until a patient had uncontrollable symptoms or showed obvious signs of joint destruction and disability. Aggressive therapy, at that time, was defined as the use of methotrexate, gold compounds, and **antimalarials.** These drugs were more effective than NSAIDs, but had higher rates of serious side effects.

Antimalarials

Drugs normally used to treat malaria but that are sometimes effective in the treatment of rheumatoid arthritis. The most commonly used antimalarial is hydroxychloroquine sulfate (Plaquenil).

Over time, research revealed that delaying aggressive treatment resulted in joint destruction and disability in patients with RA. In fact, several studies showed that a majority of the joint destruction in RA occurs in the first two years after the onset of the disease. As a result of these studies, in the 1990s physicians concentrated on limiting the destruction of joints by treating patients with more effective drugs much earlier in the course of their disease. Methotrexate and sulfasalazine were considered first-line treatment during this decade.

Since then, the introduction of the tumor necrosis factor (TNF) inhibitors—such as Remicade, Enbrel, and Humira—has changed the treatment paradigm yet again. Physicians and patients now expect better control of pain and stiffness, as well as decreased disability as a result of RA. For the first time, a significant number of patients are achieving remission. Physicians noticed that there was a difference in the rate of remission between those patients who had been treated with TNF inhibitors early in their disease and those who had started TNF inhibitors after their disease was well established. In some studies, the difference in remission rate between the early-treated and late-treated patients was three- or fourfold. This information has encouraged physicians to identify patients with RA early and to treat them aggressively with TNF inhibitors to maximize the chance of disease remission and decrease the chance of early joint destruction.

Disease remission is not disease cure, however. The RA is always there, but is suppressed by the medication only as long as you take it. Patients who have achieved disease remission and then stopped taking their medication, for example, have found that their disease often returns. You can think about your arthritis medications in much the same way you would think about medications for high blood pressure or diabetes. They might work very well, but they work only as long as you take them. Unfortunately, when these patients who stopped taking their RA medications were placed back on their treatment regimens, many were unable to achieve remission again.

If you are on a treatment regimen and it is controlling your symptoms, stick with it as long as you can: Don't tamper with success. If you believe the medication is causing problems, discuss your concerns with your physician before deciding to stop taking the drug. Your physician may be able to improve your symptoms by changing the route of administration, altering the dose of the medication, or changing to another medication altogether.

If you are on a treatment regimen and it is controlling your symptoms, stick with it as long as you can: Don't tamper with success.

I have had periods of remission. I believe this is due to medication. When my medication is cut, I get back flare-ups of the arthritis. Weather changes in the fall and spring also can cause flare ups.

—Jim

Treatment of Rheumatoid Arthritis: General Principles

PART FIVE

Medications for Rheumatoid Arthritis

What are nonsteroidal anti-inflammatory drugs?

What are disease-modifying antirheumatic drugs?

What should I know about corticosteroids?

More . . .

36. What are nonsteroidal anti-inflammatory drugs?

Nonsteroidal anti-inflammatory drugs (NSAIDs) are medications that reduce fever, pain, and inflammation. They include a large group of anti-inflammatory agents that work by inhibiting the production of **prostaglandins** (chemicals in the body that cause inflammation). As their name indicates, these drugs do not contain steroids such as prednisone, nor do they contain narcotics. NSAIDs are widely used as painkillers and as therapies for arthritis. Examples of NSAIDs include aspirin, ibuprofen, naproxen, ketoprofen, piroxicam, sulindac, choline subsalicylate, diflunisal, fenoprofen, indomethacin, meclofenamate salsalate, tolmetin, magnesium salicylate, and nabumetone, to name just a few.

Prostaglandins

Chemicals that produce pain and inflammation.

Acetaminophen (brand name: Tylenol) is not an NSAID. It has a different chemical composition and does not cause the same side effects as the NSAIDs—that is, it won't irritate your stomach the way that NSAIDs such as aspirin, naproxen sodium, or even ibuprofen sometimes can.

NSAIDs are considered safe medications. In fact, many—such as ibuprofen and aspirin—are available without a prescription (over the counter). Even so, they can cause ill effects in some people who take them. In particular, NSAIDs can cause ulcers, gastrointestinal bleeding, rashes, kidney problems, and liver dysfunction. These problems usually occur in people who take doses higher than the recommended range or who take these medications for a long time, although side effects can sometimes occur after taking a single dose in the recommended range.

As mentioned earlier, the NSAIDs work by affecting the prostaglandins, which cause inflammation in the body. Unfortunately, the same group of chemicals is involved in the stomach; thus the NSAIDs tend to cause indigestion, and may even cause ulcers and bleeding in the stomach and intestines.

NSAIDs should not be used by people who have a history of stomach or intestinal ulcers, those with bleeding disorders, or those who are taking blood thinners such as heparin or warfarin (Coumadin). If you fall into one of these categories but think you need to take an NSAID, discuss it with your physician first.

NSAIDs vary in terms of their strength and side effects. As with many medications, there is a relationship between a particular NSAID's potency and its tendency to produce side effects. For this reason, you should use these drugs with care. Take the smallest possible dose that is effective, and take no more than the maximal daily dose recommended by your physician or the product's manufacturer. In some people, NSAIDs can cause allergic reactions such as rashes, lip swelling, nasal congestion, shortness of breath, or worsening of asthma symptoms. Notify your physician if you've had an allergic reaction to aspirin or any other NSAID.

While taking NSAIDs, you should notify your physician if you have any of the following symptoms, as they may indicate a drug side effect:

- Stomach pain
- Indigestion
- Nausea or vomiting
- Dark or black stool
- Weakness
- Shortness of breath
- Rash
- Swelling of the face or extremities

Before you begin taking NSAIDs regularly, your doctor may want to do some blood tests, including a complete blood count (CBC) to make sure you are not anemic. Your physician will also perform blood tests to evaluate your liver and kidney function—in rare cases, NSAIDs can cause liver and kidney

Medications for Rheumatoid Arthritis

dysfunction. These tests should be repeated every year while you're taking NSAIDs or more frequently if you are having any symptoms.

37. What are disease-modifying antirheumatic drugs?

Signs of RA have been found in the skeletal remains of Stone Age humans, and descriptions of RA have been found in the writings of doctors and healers for thousands of years. The ancient physicians understood that the disease began with pain and stiffness and progressed to increasing joint swelling, joint deformity, limitation of motion, and disability. When physicians first began to treat RA effectively, they used drugs such as salicylic acid (aspirin) and ibuprofen (Motrin.) Doctors call these drugs nonsteroidal anti-inflammatory drugs (NSAIDs). While these drugs reduced the pain, stiffness, and swelling of inflamed joints, they did little to alter the course of the disease. For many people with RA, their disease continues to progress toward disability despite the use of NSAIDs. In an effort to improve on this therapy, medical researchers looked for medications that would both treat the symptoms of RA and prevent disease progression.

Extensive clinical research led to the introduction of a group of medications that were thought to alter the course of RA—the so-called disease-modifying antirheumatic drugs (DMARDs). DMARDs improve the signs and symptoms of RA and were thought to slow the progression of joint degeneration in some patients. Their onset of action is slower than that of NSAIDs or corticosteroids; they improve symptoms of RA only after several weeks to months in some cases. In addition, DMARDs are associated with more adverse side effects than the NSAIDs.

To decide whether use of a DMARD is necessary, a physician may evaluate the condition of the patient's joints by taking x-rays of those joints that are swollen and tender. If the x-rays reveal the development of erosions or joint space narrowing, it

Table 1 The currently available DMARDs include:

Chemical name	Brand Name
Methotrexate	Rheumatrex, Trexall
Antimalarials • Hydroxychloroquine • Chloroquine	Plaquenil, Quineprox, Aralen
Sulfasalazine	Azulfidine
Leflunomide	Arava
Tumor Necrosis Factor Inhibitors	Remicade, Humira, Enbrel,
Soluble Interleukin–1 (IL–1) Receptor Therapy	Kineret
Gold Compounds	Auranofin, Solganal, Aurolate
Cytotoxic Agents • Azathioprine • Cyclophosphamide • Cyclosporine A	Imuran Cytoxan Neoral
Penicillamine	Cuprimine, Depen

is a clear indication for DMARD therapy. Physicians should not wait for these changes to occur before treating patients, however. Once a patient experiences persistent disease activity, his or her doctor should consider prescribing one of the DMARD agents.

Many factors influence which particular DMARD a physician will choose for a patient. The doctor must consider the following questions:

- How effective is this medication compared to the other DMARDs?
- Will administering a particular drug be more or less convenient for the patient?
- What are the requirements of the monitoring program for this drug?

Once a patient experiences persistent disease activity, his or her doctor should consider prescribing a disease-modifying antirheumatic drug.

Medications for Rheumatoid Arthritis

- How expensive is this drug, and what are the costs of tests to monitor the patient? Can the patient afford to pay for the DMARD?
- What is the likelihood of the patient being able to comply with this drug regimen?
- Does the patient have other medical conditions that might interfere with the effectiveness of this medication?
- Are the risks associated with the DMARD appropriate given the severity of the patient's disease?
- What is the physician's level of familiarity with this medication? Is he or she confident enough to administer it, deal with any side effects, and monitor the patient while he or she is on this drug?

You should discuss with your doctor the benefits and risks of every medication you take.

38. What should I know about corticosteroids?

Corticosteroids (or, as they are more commonly known, "steroids") are a class of medications that are often given to people with inflammatory diseases. These medications are similar to natural hormone substances that are produced by the body. Steroids help to reduce inflammation and have been used for more than 50 years to treat RA. They work by both decreasing inflammation and depressing the immune system (making it less active).

Steroids are very effective in decreasing symptoms of joint pain, swelling, and stiffness. In fact, recent studies report that taking at least three months of treatment with low-dose oral corticosteroids significantly reduces pain and joint inflammation while improving joint function. These medications can reduce your level of fatigue and rapidly improve your overall symptoms. Your doctor may prescribe steroids either to control painful flares of arthritis or to act as a "bridge" therapy until a slower-acting medication takes effect.

Steroids can be given as pills, intramuscular injections, or intravenous infusions. They can even be injected directly into inflamed joints. Names of commonly used steroid medications include betamethasone, budesonide, cortisone, dexamethasone, flunisolide, fluticasone, hydrocortisone, prednisone, prednisolone, and methylprednisolone.

Physicians often prescribe steroids for short periods (two to three months), with the objective of suppressing generalized arthritic flares or as temporary adjunctive therapy while waiting for the other medications (DMARDs or biologic agents) to exert their anti-inflammatory effects. Alternatively, physicians may prescribe steroids for longer periods (two years or more) in an attempt to modify the progression of RA and prevent destruction of the joints. For patients with severe disease, whose symptoms are not well controlled on maximal doses of NSAIDs, DMARDs, or biologic therapies, corticosteroids can be useful as chronic adjunctive therapy.

Corticosteroids often provide rapid, dramatic relief of the pain and inflammation caused by RA. Unfortunately, as with many other arthritis medications, joints often become inflamed again after corticosteroids are discontinued, unless the patient also takes DMARDs.

These serious side effects include:

- Destruction of the hip, knee, wrist, or foot joints (osteonecrosis)
- Bone thinning and weakening (osteoporosis)
- Cataracts
- Swelling caused by fluid retention (edema)
- Weight gain
- Acne
- Rounding of facial features (moon face)
- Mood swings, depression, difficulty concentrating, insomnia, anxiety, and euphoria

Medications for Rheumatoid Arthritis

Corticosteroids often provide rapid, dramatic relief of the pain and inflammation caused by RA. Unfortunately, long-term use of steroids can have serious side effects.

- Easy bruising
- Increased risk of infection from immune suppression
- Elevated blood pressure
- Elevated blood sugar levels (diabetes)
- Muscle weakness
- Glaucoma

As with any medication, you must weigh the risks of taking a steroid against the benefits it offers. Steroids' side effects usually occur when higher dosages are given over a long period of time (weeks to months); most people who use steroids for only a short period of time do not suffer side effects. You should discuss the benefits and risks of taking steroids with your physician before filling the prescription. A good goal to keep in mind is summarized in this way: the smallest possible dose, for the shortest duration of time. Patients with RA frequently take small doses of steroids, but for long periods of time.

One potentially serious side effect of long-term steroid use is adrenal suppression. Under normal circumstances, the body's adrenal system produces cortisol (a naturally produced steroid); the brain, in turn, monitors the cortisol levels in the bloodstream. The brain cannot tell the difference between the body's own cortisol and the steroid medication provided by the doctor, however. Thus the adrenal gland, because it is no longer called upon to produce natural steroids, may shut down. Over time, a person who is taking high doses of steroids may become unable to rapidly produce natural steroids from his or her adrenal gland. If your doctor is uncertain about whether you will be able to taper off steroids after a long period of treatment owing to adrenal suppression, the doctor might recommend that you take a cortrosyn stimulation test. This test can determine whether your adrenal glands still retain the ability to produce cortisol.

If you take steroids for a long time, your doctor may recommend that you take a larger dose of steroids before you undergo surgery, after a serious accident, or in a stressful situation. This larger dose is intended to compensate for your body's inability to increase its natural steroid production to the level necessary to tolerate these stresses. The increased steroid levels during stress allow the body to maintain blood pressure and normal heart function. When you and your doctor determine that you no longer require the steroids, your physician will gradually lower the dose you're taking, allowing your own adrenal gland to slowly increase its production to normal levels.

This phenomenon explains why it is so important that you continue taking steroid medications regularly and do not stop their use abruptly. Even if you don't have any refills left on your prescription, it is a good idea to check with your doctor and confirm that the doctor intended for you to stop treatment. If you have any doubts about what you should do, ask your doctor.

There are a few things you can do to limit the side effects of steroids—specifically, go on a low-calorie, low-salt diet; make sure that you consume an adequate amount of vitamin D and calcium; and get enough weight-bearing exercise. You should discuss all of these issues with your physician, who can make specific recommendations about diet and exercise. In addition, your doctor may prescribe other medications that will help prevent bone loss, such as Actonel, Fosamax, Boniva, or calcitonin. Patients with and without osteoporosis risk factors who are taking low-dose prednisone should also undergo bone densitometry tests to assess their fracture risk.

Corticosteroids—I have had cortisone injections in the knees, hands, and the shoulders. They work for about a 30-day period. Just enough time to get me through the flare up.

—Jim

Prednisone was my best friend for many years. I was usually prescribed a low dose in combination with other medications. Any time I had a bad flare up—my right hand could really swell to the point where I couldn't use it. I could count on a steroid packet to give me relief within about 24 hours. But I also knew that long term use of steroids can have serious side effects. Despite this, it was worth it to get rid of my symptoms.

—Nona

39. What is methotrexate?

Methotrexate is a very commonly prescribed RA medication and is the most popular of the disease-modifying antirheumatic drugs (DMARDs). It is also known by its brand name, Rheumatrex (Stada Pharmaceuticals).

Methotrexate is classified as an antimetabolite drug, which means it is capable of blocking the metabolism of cells. It is particularly effective in suppressing rapidly dividing cells, such as those found in the inflamed joints of people with RA. This drug is effective in both reducing the signs and symptoms of RA and slowing disease progression and joint damage. Its effects start within weeks after you first begin to take methotrexate, but can take months to reach their full effectiveness. Methotrexate's ability to improve symptoms depends on how high a dose you take. Ordinarily, doctors prescribe a low dose initially, between 7.5 and 15 milligrams per week. This dose is increased until symptoms improve, which may take several months. People rarely tolerate doses higher than 20 to 25 milligrams.

Methotrexate has many positive attributes:

- It is effective in most patients with RA (70% of patients have some response).
- It begins to work within four to six weeks.
- It has fewer side effects than some other DMARDs.
- It is well tolerated for long periods of time (the majority of patients will still be on the drug after five years).
- It is easy to administer (weekly pills or injections).
- It is relatively inexpensive.

Methotrexate can be taken as pills or can be given as a subcutaneous (under the skin) injection. Some people may experience nausea after taking methotrexate orally. Taking the medication as a subcutaneous injection seems to reduce or eliminate this problem. Giving the methotrexate as an injection in the skin allows for the use of a small needle (the size of an insulin needle), and a relatively painless injection. Intramuscular injections can hurt a bit. However, many people find they can tolerate higher dose of methotrexate when it is given by an intramuscular injection, because it seems to cause less nausea.

Common side effects of methotrexate include nausea, stomach upset, hair loss, and stomatitis. Stomatitis is an inflammation of the mucous lining of any of the structures in the mouth, which may involve the cheeks, gums, tongue, lips, and roof or floor of the mouth. People who experience this side effect usually don't have visible ulcers in their mouth, but they may have a lot of pain and difficulty eating.

Rare and more serious side effects of methotrexate are those affecting the liver, lungs, and bone marrow. The liver can become inflamed as a result of methotrexate, a condition known as hepatitis. Prolonged exposure in some people can result in the liver becoming filled with nonfunctioning fibrous tissue, a condition called hepatic cirrhosis. The incidence of real toxicity is probably on the order of 1 in 1000 patients over a five-year treatment period. Your doctor will monitor your blood tests to make sure you aren't developing problems with your blood or your liver if you take methotrexate.

Patients who take methotrexate can also develop fibrosis of the lungs, an uncommon but potentially fatal complication known as interstitial pneumonitis. The risk factors for methotrexate-related lung disease are not well understood, but may include preexisting lung disease or an abnormal chest radiograph.

Medications for Rheumatoid Arthritis

Platelet

An irregular, disc-shaped element in the blood that assists in blood clotting.

Methotrexate can also suppress the production of blood cells and **platelets** in the bone marrow. Because of these risks, before you start taking this medication, your physician should order baseline studies of your blood, liver, and lungs to confirm that you're not at high risk for developing these complications. Some specific studies you should have before beginning methotrexate therapy include the following tests:

- A complete blood count (CBC)
- Liver function chemistries and tests for hepatitis B and C
- Serum creatinine level (a measure of kidney function)
- Chest x-ray and pulmonary function tests

Once you begin taking methotrexate, your doctor should order a CBC and tests of liver and kidney function every four to eight weeks.

Folic acid (a B vitamin), in a dose of 1000 micrograms per day, is usually prescribed for people who take methotrexate in an effort to prevent many of the side effects associated with this medication. Some people will do well on methotrexate without folic acid; of course, given that the folic acid doesn't decrease the efficacy of the methotrexate, it seems like a wise precaution to take it just in case side effects do occur. Occasionally, higher doses of folic acid are used in conjunction with methotrexate, or other forms of folic acid such as folinic acid are used.

Methotrexate can be combined safely with nearly every other FDA-approved DMARD for RA, including NSAIDs, sulfasalazine, hydroxychloroquine, leflunomide, and tumor necrosis factor (TNF) inhibitors. No unexpected toxicities have been observed in medical studies when methotrexate was combined with one of these DMARDs.

Not all patients are good candidates for methotrexate therapy. If you have problems with your liver, kidneys, or bone marrow, you should notify your physician before you begin taking methotrexate. People who have chronic obstructive pulmonary disease (COPD, also known as emphysema), renal insufficiency, or acute or chronic liver disease; people who abuse alcohol; people who are malnourished; and people who have some blood diseases may also be at a higher risk for experiencing methotrexate's side effects.

I've been on methotrexate since 1993. This medication works for me in the pill form. I do have flare ups when they cut back on the number of pills or when the weather (seasons) changes. I have blood work done on a monthly basis.

—Jim

40. What is leflunomide?

Leflunomide is a new DMARD. It was approved by the FDA as a treatment for rheumatoid arthritis in October 1998, and is sold under the name Arava in the United States. This drug has a different chemical structure than other DMARDs and a unique mechanism of action for improving RA symptoms.

Leflunomide is an effective treatment for RA symptoms. In fact, medical studies demonstrate that it is as effective as methotrexate and sulfasalazine in treating the signs and symptoms of RA. Improvement of symptoms usually begins four to eight weeks after a person starts taking leflunomide. Like the other DMARDs, leflunomide also slows the joint destruction caused by RA.

Most patients with RA can tolerate treatment with leflunomide. In fact, in studies comparing the tolerability of various DMARDs, leflunomide has been shown to have fewer withdrawals from medical trials than methotrexate and sulfasalazine.

Because of its effectiveness, tolerability, and unique mechanism of action, leflunomide represents a viable alternative for

Because of its effectiveness, tolerability, and unique mechanism of action, leflunomide represents a viable alternative for patients who have failed or are intolerant to methotrexate.

patients who have failed or are intolerant to methotrexate. Interestingly, leflunomide can be given to patients who are already taking methotrexate but do not have an adequate response to the latter medication. If the patient has no preexisting liver disease and if liver function tests are monitored on a monthly basis, then leflunomide and methotrexate can be combined safely.

Leflunomide has been associated with liver function abnormalities that improve after patients stop the medication. It can also cause stomach upset, diarrhea, and hair loss. Leflunomide can affect the development of fetuses, so women of childbearing age should be made aware of this risk and advised to use birth control while on this medication. Unlike other DMARDs, however, leflunomide treatment does not appear to be associated with an increased risk for infection.

Your doctor should perform regular blood tests while you're on leflunomide. These tests should include a complete blood count and liver function tests every two weeks for the first month while you are taking leflunomide, and then the same tests on a monthly basis thereafter.

41. What is sulfasalazine?

Sulfasalazine (brand name: Azulfidine) is an effective DMARD that is used in the treatment of RA. This drug is created from the combination of salicylic acid (the active ingredient in aspirin) and sulfapyridine (an antibiotic). It is given by mouth and is available in the form of time-release tablets. Like the other DMARDs, sulfasalazine has been shown not only to reduce the signs and symptoms of RA, but also to slow or halt joint destruction.

Rheumatologists are unsure of how this medication works to improve symptoms, but studies have demonstrated that more than half of all patients treated with sulfasalazine have improvements in their pain symptoms. Like the other

DMARDs, sulfasalazine may take several months before it helps to reduce the pain and swelling of RA. Rheumatologists reserve sulfasalazine for use in early, milder cases of RA or as an alternative to methotrexate in patients with liver disease. The usual dose is 2 to 3 grams per day, with pills being taken twice daily.

Sulfasalazine may be used in combination therapy with NSAIDs and other DMARDs for more active RA. Because this drug is a combination of aspirin and a sulfur-containing antibiotic, people with sulfa or aspirin allergies should not use it.

Sulfasalazine can cause side effects that are severe enough to stop treatment in as many as 22% of patients. The most common side effects include allergic reactions, stomach upset, skin rashes, abnormal blood cell counts, and liver problems. To monitor for these problems, tests of liver function and blood cell counts should be performed every one to three months depending on dose.

42. What is Plaquenil?

Plaquenil (hydroxychloroquine) is an antimalarial drug that is commonly prescribed to treat RA, systemic lupus erythematosus, and some other rheumatic diseases. This class of medications has a long history. Antimalarial medications that are also useful in treating arthritis were first developed from the bark of the Peruvian cinchona tree.

Plaquenil is one of a group of slow-acting medications used to treat RA. People who take this medication must realize that it will take a few weeks to a few months before they see improvement in their symptoms. In my own practice, when I ask people to start this medication, I typically have them schedule their next appointment for two months because this is a good time interval to check for improvement. Because the benefits of Plaquenil take so long to become apparent, some patients may find it necessary to take it in conjunction with other medications that work in the interim period.

Plaquenil is generally well tolerated. The most common side effect is upset stomach, although Plaquenil doesn't contribute to stomach ulcer formation (unlike NSAIDs and corticosteroids). A skin rash can occur in patients who are allergic to the medication. Sometimes dizziness, blurred vision, or headache may occur. When the drug is taken over a long period of time, bleaching of the hair or gray discoloration of the skin can occur. Blood problems are very uncommon with this medication, so Plaquenil requires very little monitoring of blood tests.

There is a very remote possibility that Plaquenil may cause pigment deposition in the retina (the back of the eye) and lead to vision loss in some patients. Although the chance of this side effect occurring while you are taking Plaquenil at the prescribed dosage is very remote, it is still a good idea to see an eye doctor. The first visit to the eye doctor should be scheduled after about six months of treatment with the medication, and then annually thereafter. The eye doctor will check carefully for any evidence of pigment deposition in the macula (the central part of the retina) and perform other tests to look for any subtle change in vision. The eye doctor may also give you an Amsler Grid, a useful tool for monitoring your central visual field at home. This test is important for detecting early and sometimes subtle visual changes.

Plaquenil has the potential to cause damage to an unborn child, which is an important concern for women of childbearing age who take this drug. The conventional advice is that this medication, like many other arthritis medications, should be stopped prior to becoming pregnant. Small series of case reports in the medical literature reporting on women who took these medications during pregnancy and had healthy babies suggest that Plaquenil is safe for use during pregnancy. Nevertheless, the risks and benefits must be carefully weighed, and you should definitely discuss this issue with your doctor.

In general, Plaquenil is well tolerated and is ideally suited for people with mild RA. It is also frequently used in combination with other medications such as methotrexate.

I've been taking Plaquenil along with my methotrexate since 1993. It's important to have your eyes examined once a year while you're taking Plaquenil. I have had no side effects from this medication.

—Jim

43. What are tumor necrosis factor inhibitors?

Tumor necrosis factor (TNF) inhibitors are a new class of biologic therapies that have changed the face of rheumatology over the past decade. TNF inhibitor therapy can lead to dramatic improvements in RA symptoms and prevent joint destruction. Unlike the typical arthritis drugs, which tend to be composed of small molecules, TNF inhibitors are complex antibodies (proteins) that are directed against the chemical signal that causes inflammation in your body.

Tumor necrosis factor alpha (TNF-α) is a chemical that is produced by some of the white blood cells in your body during the immune response. It stimulates inflammation, which in turn helps to fight infection and repair damaged tissues in your body. In RA, the inflammatory process mediated by TNF-α gets out of control and results in the pain, redness, and swelling that is characteristic of RA. Scientific studies have shown that TNF-α is found in large quantities in the swollen joints of people with RA.

TNF inhibitors work by binding to the naturally produced TNF-α molecules in the joints and bloodstream. When the TNF inhibitor medication binds to TNF-α molecules, it renders them ineffective and removes them from the bloodstream. Without the stimulation of the TNF-α, the inflammation decreases and symptoms are reduced. In addition to reduc-

Tumor necrosis factor (TNF) inhibitors have changed the face of rheumatology over the past decade. TNF inhibitor therapy can lead to dramatic improvements in RA symptoms and prevent joint destruction.

Medications for Rheumatoid Arthritis

ing the signs and symptoms of RA, extensive medical studies have shown that TNF inhibitors can slow—or even stop completely—joint damage.

TNF inhibitors are administered either through intravenous infusion or by a subcutaneous injection. The time between injections can range from weeks to months, depending on the specific agent and the severity of your disease.

Currently, three TNF inhibitors are approved in the United States for the treatment of RA: infliximab (Remicade), etanercept (Enbrel), and adalimumab (Humira). Several more TNF inhibitors are currently being reviewed by the FDA. All of these therapies are expensive, however, so you should find out which agents your insurance will cover and discuss this issue with your physician before beginning therapy.

TNF-α inhibitors suppress the immune system and can place you at higher risk for infections. Usually, these infections are minor infections of the upper respiratory or urinary tract and can be easily managed with antibiotics. Unfortunately, some life-threatening infections and deaths from infections have been associated TNF-α inhibitor use. Therefore, if you are taking one of these medications, you should not ignore signs of infection, such as fever, cough, headache, weakness, and abdominal or back pain, as they may be signs of a serious problem. Some physicians tell their patients that while they are taking TNF-α inhibitors, they are "not allowed to have a cold or flu!" That is, patients shouldn't assume that a mild cough or fever is "just a cold" but rather should contact their physician and make sure they are medically evaluated to prevent serious or life-threatening infections.

Cases of lymphoma and tuberculosis have also been associated with the use of all TNF-α inhibitors. The risk of lymphoma is discussed in Question 30, and the risk of infections is discussed in Question 27.

Over the past seven years I've used all three of these anti-TNF drugs. The first one I tried was Remicade. This product is given intravenously over a period of about 2–3 hours. It was such a production—I really didn't like it. It made me feel like a cancer patient receiving chemotherapy. This was a very depressing stage for me. In addition, the results after many treatments were not satisfactory. The next anti-TNF I tried was Humira. Humira is a medication that you can inject yourself, sort of like insulin. Unfortunately, a few hours after my first injection I developed a severe allergic reaction. I was covered in a rash from head to toe. It was incredibly uncomfortable—hot and itchy. My doctor had to put me on a heavy dose of steroids to counter the reaction. It took over a week for the rash to subside. Finally, about a year ago, my doctor suggested that I try Enbrel, another of the anti-TNF drugs. I was so depressed when he told me this because again I would have to give myself an injection once a week—I had been through a year of injections with methotrexate and never got comfortable injecting myself. I felt I really had no choice because of my worsening symptoms. So I gave it a try and now a year later I can say the results have been fantastic. No more flare ups and very little swelling at all in my hands. Another great thing about Enbrel is that it comes in syringes that are pre-filled for you. This took away the anxiety I had with the whole process of giving myself methotrexate injections. I had to measure the right amount and was afraid of giving myself too much or too little. My rheumatologist told me that is not unusual for someone to try different anti-TNF medications till they find the one that works. Some people respond to Remicade and would rather have an intravenous infusion every eight weeks than inject themselves every week or two. Others prefer the autonomy of being able to inject themselves and not bother with spending several hours at the doctor's office. For others, it is an issue of which product their insurance will pay for. You should discuss these issues with your doctor before starting one of these anti-TNF agents.

—Nona

44. My doctor wants me to try a new drug called abatacept. What is it?

Abatacept (brand name: Orenica) is the first in a new class of biologic agents used in the treatment of RA. The members of this class are collectively called co-stimulation modulators.

T cells play an important role in your immune system by fighting off viruses, bacteria, and other disease-causing agents. A normal immune system leaves healthy body tissues alone. Unfortunately in RA, for reasons that are not clear, T cells become activated and attack healthy tissues. Activated T cells play a central role in the inflammatory cascade, leading to the joint inflammation and destruction characteristic of RA. Abatacept has the ability to block the activation of the T cells, thereby decreasing the signs and symptoms of RA.

Abatacept is approved by the FDA for treatment of people with moderately to severely active RA who have shown an inadequate response to one of the DMARDs (e.g., methotrexate, leflunomide, or hydroxychloroquine) or TNF inhibitors (etanercept, adalimumab, or infliximab). It is commonly prescribed along with methotrexate or other DMARDs, but should not be administered with a TNF inhibitor owing to the increased risk of side effects with this combination.

Similar to infliximab, abatacept is given as an intravenous infusion. Whereas infliximab takes two hours to infuse, however, abatacept can be administered over 30 minutes. Abatacept needs to be administered every month.

Potential side effects of abatacept include allergic reactions, an increased risk for infections, and cancer. In particular, treatment with abatacept can make you more prone to getting infections or make any infection you already have worse. It is important to tell your doctor if you think you have any infections before beginning therapy with abatacept. If you develop a fever, cough, chills, or pain or burning when you urinate during your treatment with abatacept, you should see your doctor immediately or go to the emergency room to be evaluated.

45. What are gold compounds?

Gold compounds have been used to treat diseases for centuries. The ancient Chinese thought ingesting gold would prolong life and increase vitality. In Europe in the sixteenth century, gold compounds were used to treat epilepsy and depression. In the late nineteenth century microbiologists discovered that gold inhibited the growth of tubercle bacilli, the organism responsible for tuberculosis. In 1929 doctors began using gold to treat RA, because of the mistaken notion that RA was caused by a tuberculosis infection. Though an infectious cause for RA has never been proven, the use of gold compounds was noted to have a positive effect on the symptoms of RA. As a result its use was continued, even without an understanding of how it worked.

Chrysotherapy or aurotherapy are terms used to describe treatment with gold compounds. Gold salts accumulate slowly in the body and, over time, reduce inflammation. Several injectable forms of gold and one oral form of gold have been used to treat RA. Initially injections are given every week. After a few months the interval between injections is gradually increased to two weeks, and eventually monthly. Treatment with gold compounds can lead to injuries of the bone marrow and kidneys. Therefore, an examination of the blood and urine are necessary before each injection. These test results had to be reviewed by the doctor before the injection, so this made treatment more expensive, and caused people to spend more time in the office. Treatment with gold injections is a slow process. Even trying to decide if gold treatment is successful takes a long time. It was not unusual to continue this treatment for four to six months before a decision could be reached regarding its effectiveness for that person. Great patience was called for!

Medications for Rheumatoid Arthritis

More recently gold became available in capsule form (aura-nofin). Although this form of treatment is much more convenient than injectable forms of gold, it doesn't work as well, and it has more side effects, such as hair thinning, decreased appetite, nausea and diarrhea. Gold treatments frequently help RA, but most people are off the medication in two years or less because of a high level of side effects. Common side effects of gold treatment include abnormal blood counts, protein in the urine, and skin rashes. Other common side effects include sore tongue, sore gums, or disturbances of taste sensation.

Today, gold treatment is very seldom used for RA. It has largely been replaced by more effective and better tolerated medications.

46. What is rituximab?

Rituximab (pronounced "ri-TUX-i-mab") is an antibody that was originally created in the laboratory. It is designed to interact with B cells, which are a type of white blood cells that play a role in the initiation and development of RA. Rituximab (brand name: Rituxan) decreases the number of B cells in the circulation. In fact, people who take rituximab have demonstrated near-complete depletion of B cells in their bloodstream within two weeks of taking the first dose of medication. Most people showed a sustained peripheral B-cell depletion that lasted for at least six months. The B cells returned to their normal level gradually thereafter. Plasma cells (the cells that make antibodies) are not depleted by rituximab, however; likewise, levels of the antibodies that are necessary to fight infections do not decline.

Rituximab was originally sold as a novel treatment for lymphoma (a cancer of the lymph nodes). Patients with both lymphoma and RA who underwent treatment with rituximab noticed that their RA symptoms were significantly improved after treatment, leading to further investigation of this antibody as a treatment for RA. Rituximab is now indicated for the treatment of patients with RA who have shown an inadequate response to previous treatment with one or more TNF inhibitor therapies.

Rituximab is given to patients as two intravenous infusions, whose delivery is separated by two weeks. This course of treatment is repeated every six to nine months. The dose of rituximab will be different for different patients. The dose that is used may depend on a number of things, including your weight.

This medication should be administered only by or under the immediate supervision of your doctor. Rituximab is given in combination with methotrexate, which boosts the effectiveness of both treatments. Additionally, before each infusion, it has been recommended that methylprednisolone be given. This steroid decreases the likelihood of an infusion reaction, and probably contributes to the effectiveness of the treatment as well.

Like many other arthritis drugs, rituximab should be given only after you have discussed all of the risks and benefits associated with its use. For many people, being treated with this antibody can result in significant improvements in their RA symptoms. Unfortunately, there are also side effects that anyone contemplating treatment should discuss with their physician:

- Some patients may experience an allergic reaction during the infusion of rituximab. This reaction can be as mild as minor itching and hives or as serious as low blood pressure and difficulty breathing. Because of this possibility, rituximab is administered with corticosteroids, which tend to blunt any allergic reaction.
- Rituximab may decrease the number of white blood cells, red blood cells, and platelets. If you experience a decrease in these blood constituents, you may be at increased risk for anemia, infections, and bleeding.

- Any drug that depresses the immune system puts the person treated at increased risk for infection. People treated with rituximab have been noted to have an increase in infections of the sinuses, lungs, and urinary tract. If you are taking rituximab (or any other drug that suppresses the immune system), you are also at risk for serious infections that can result in hospitalization or death if not treated immediately. Consequently, if you experience fever or chills, cough, shortness of breath, sore throat, or pain or difficulty passing urine, you should contact your doctor immediately or go to the emergency room.

PART SIX

Testing for Rheumatoid Arthritis

My doctor told me I had to get a test for rheumatoid factor. What is that?

How accurate is the rheumatoid factor test?

What is a sedimentation rate?

More . . .

47. My doctor told me I had to get a test for rheumatoid factor. What is that?

The test for rheumatoid factor (RF) is ordered when you have symptoms of RA, such as stiffness in your joints for a long time in the morning, swelling, nodules under your skin, and evidence on x-rays of swollen joints and loss of cartilage and bone. Rheumatoid factor is an antibody that is measurable in the blood. Although antibodies are normal proteins in our blood and are important parts of our immune system, the RF antibody is not usually present in the normal individual (although it can be found in 1% to 2% of healthy people). When healthy people have RF, it is usually present in only a small amount. The incidence of RF in healthy people increases with age, such that as many as 20% of people older than age 65 have an elevated RF level.

Approximately 80% to 90% of patients with RA have high amounts of RF in their blood. This antibody can usually be detected after a person starts noticing joint pain and stiffness. The amount of RF in the bloodstream increases slowly after symptoms first occur. That is, the incidence of RF increases with the duration of disease in RA. Commonly, only 33% of people who have had RA for three months have detectable amounts of RF; one year after the onset of the disease, the incidence of elevated RF levels jumps to 75%.

High levels (titers) of RF are associated with more severe RA and a higher mortality risk in patients with RA than individuals without this disease. In addition, RF is known to be abundant in the synovium and cartilage of patients with RA. High levels of RF have also been associated with an increased tendency to develop the non-joint complications of RA, such as rheumatoid nodules and rheumatoid lung disease. There is a much lower prevalence of RF in patients with juvenile RA.

A blood test is used to detect the presence of RF. It requires a small blood sample, which is usually drawn from your arm in the doctor's office or a clinical laboratory.

48. How accurate is the rheumatoid factor test?

Rheumatoid arthritis cannot be diagnosed with a blood test alone. The RF test is helpful in making the diagnosis of RA, but it isn't foolproof. Notably, this test produces both false-positive and false-negative results.

With a false-positive result, a positive RF test doesn't necessarily mean that you have RA. Many reasons other than the presence of RA can cause a person to test positive for RF. For example, the following autoimmune diseases are associated with elevated RF levels:

- Sjögren's syndrome
- Systemic lupus erythematosus
- Scleroderma
- Polymyositis/dermatomyositis
- Mixed connective tissue disease

A variety of infections may also be associated with a positive RF test:

- Bacterial endocarditis (an infection of the lining of the heart)
- Osteomyelitis (an infection of the bone)
- Tuberculosis
- Syphilis
- Hepatitis (inflammation of the liver)
- Mononucleosis

Finally, the following conditions may also produce a positive test for RF:

- Diffuse interstitial pulmonary fibrosis
- Liver cirrhosis
- Sarcoidosis
- Multiple vaccinations

Rheumatoid arthritis cannot be diagnosed with a blood test alone. The rheumatoid factor test is helpful in making the diagnosis of RA, but it isn't foolproof.

Testing for Rheumatoid Arthritis

- Lipemia (a large amount of fat in the blood)
- Medication reaction (e.g., methyldopa, a blood pressure drug, can increase the amount of RF detected by the test)
- Improper handling of the blood specimen
- An organ transplant from a person not related to you

Several conditions are characterized by painful swollen joints but are *not* associated with elevated RF levels:

Ankylosing

Crooked or bent; refers to stiffening of the joint.

- Osteoarthritis
- **Ankylosing** spondylitis
- Gout
- Psoriatic arthritis
- Reactive arthritis (also known as Reiter's syndrome)

With a false-negative result, a negative RF test result does not always mean that you do not have RA. Perhaps it is too early in the progression of your disease to detect RF, or you are in a remission phase, or you have a type of RA that occurs without elevated RF levels. In fact, as many as 20% of patients with RA remain negative for RF (also known as "seronegative rheumatoid arthritis") throughout the course of their disease. For these reasons, if a person tests negative for RF yet continues to have arthritic symptoms, the RF test may need to be repeated. Conversely, if the RF test is positive and the diagnosis of RA is established, there is little benefit in repeating the RF test.

The uncertainty associated with the RF test results is why your doctor needs to take a thorough history and physical exam in addition to administering tests like those for RF, antinuclear antibodies, and x-rays, before he or she can make a definitive diagnosis of RA.

49. What is a sedimentation rate?

A sedimentation rate is a blood test that is commonly performed on patients with RA. This test is also sometimes referred to as a "sed rate" or an **erythrocyte sedimentation rate (ESR)**. The sedimentation rate measures how fast the red blood cells (erythrocytes) settle (become sediment) in the bottom of a glass tube.

RA is characterized by inflammation of the joints and other tissues. When inflammation occurs, the body produces many proteins that help fight infection and repair injured tissues. The more inflammation the body experiences, the more proteins it produces. These extra proteins cause the red blood cells to settle faster in the bottom of a glass tube. Therefore, it can be inferred that the more rapidly the red blood cells drop, the more inflammation (that is, RA) is present in the body. The sed rate tends to reflect the clinical disease activity and to parallel such symptoms as morning stiffness and fatigue. Joint examination by the physician is far more useful in assessing the amount of joint inflammation (called **synovitis**).

A sed rate is performed on a sample of blood. Blood is drawn from the patient's vein, usually from the inside of the elbow or the back of the hand. A small amount of anticoagulant is added to the blood sample to keep the blood cells from clotting. The blood cells are placed in a special glass tube that is calibrated with millimeter markings on the side, and the blood is allowed to settle for one hour. After the hour has elapsed, the level of the top of the red blood cell layer is measured and recorded. The normal sedimentation rate is 0 to 15 millimeters per hour for men and 0 to 20 millimeters per hour for women. In healthy people who are more than 60 years old, the normal sedimentation rate can be slightly elevated.

Effective treatment of RA will decrease the amount of inflammation and, therefore, lower the sed rate. A physician may check a patient's sed rate frequently to see whether the treatment is working successfully. Keep in mind that a normal sed rate doesn't mean that you are cured and no longer need treatment for RA.

Erythrocyte sedimentation rate (ESR)

A diagnostic test for inflammatory diseases that measures the rate at which red blood cells settle out from a well-mixed specimen of blood.

Synovitis

Inflammation of the synovium.

Testing for Rheumatoid Arthritis

A normal sedimentation rate doesn't mean that you are cured and no longer need treatment for RA.

50. What does the sedimentation rate mean?

The sedimentation rate ("sed rate") is not a perfect test, and using it can pose a challenge for physicians. An elevated sed rate is understood by physicians to be neither sensitive nor specific for RA. A highly sensitive test for RA would give a positive result for *all* people with RA; a highly specific test would give a positive result for *only* those people with RA and for no one else. A very sensitive and specific test would be a boon to patients and physicians alike. With a single blood test, the physician could make the diagnosis and start treatment. Unfortunately, such a test does not currently exist.

The sed rate is often elevated in RA, but not universally so. In fact, only 60% of people with RA have an elevated sed rate. Additionally, if a person has an elevated sed rate, it does not mean that individual has RA because an elevated sed rate is a nonspecific finding. In other words, it does not identify any particular disease, but merely indicates that inflammation is occurring in the body somewhere. Diseases other than RA that can produce an elevated sed rate include polymyalgia rheumatica, systemic lupus erythematosus, ulcerative colitis, heart attack, certain cancers, leukemia, tuberculosis, and other bacterial and viral infections. A sed rate can even be increased during a normal pregnancy.

Patients often wonder why they need a blood test that is so nonspecific and does not appear to help make the diagnosis of RA. Physicians understand that the sed rate sometimes helps to confirm an uncertain diagnosis or enables the physician to better monitor the disease activity. A new patient who presents with some joint or muscle pain but has a normal sed rate is less likely to have RA. A patient with established RA who complains of increased pain in his knee might be having a flare of his RA that will require an increase of medication or might be suffering from the effects of minor trauma. An elevated sed rate in this situation would suggest an increase in inflammation due to worsening RA. The physician could then treat the person with antirheumatic drugs with greater confidence and a better chance of improvement.

The sed rate test shouldn't be ordered as part of an annual physical examination, unless the doctor has a strong suspicion that the patient is sick. A sed rate in this setting is analogous to a low-grade fever. A low-grade fever isn't normal, but the list of its possible causes is almost endless and can result in needless worry and fruitless searches for a cause. In most situations, the C-reactive protein (CRP) test is a better option than the sedimentation rate for identifying RA; the CRP test is discussed in more detail in Question 57.

51. What is a complete blood count?

A complete blood count (CBC) is a measurement of the components of the blood. This test can help your doctor both diagnose disease and monitor the safety of any treatments administered for a disease. The CBC is also called a blood count, a hemogram, or a CBC with differential.

While many other blood tests measure the amount of a particular drug, chemical, or protein in your blood, the CBC checks the blood cells themselves. It measures the numbers of different types of blood cells as well as their sizes, shapes, color, and other characteristics. Abnormal results in the CBC can reflect problems with the amount of fluid in your body (such as dehydration) or loss of blood. This test can also give an indication of the amounts of iron and some vitamins in your body. It can show abnormalities in the production, life span, and destruction of blood cells. Finally, the CBC can highlight acute or chronic infection, allergies, and problems with clotting.

Having a CBC will take just a few minutes of your time. No special preparation or fasting before the test is necessary. A CBC utilizes a small sample of blood that is usually drawn from a vein in your arm or the back of your hand. The test carries no risk of getting AIDS, hepatitis, or any other blood-borne disease. The blood sample is sent to the lab, where automated machines rapidly count the cell types.

Some of the constituents of the blood that are measured in the CBC include white blood cells (WBC), red blood cells (RBC), and platelets (PLT).

White Blood Cell Count

White blood cells are part of your immune system and help the body fight off infections. Normal values for the WBC count range between 4000 and 10,000 cells per cubic milliliter (cmm). A high WBC count could suggest inflammation, which might be due to RA. However, infections, stress, exercise, and medications such as steroids may also temporarily elevate the WBC count. A low WBC count may result from certain blood diseases, bone marrow failure, and some auto-immune diseases. Some of the medications used to treat RA can lead to low WBC counts, especially the disease-modifying antirheumatic drugs (DMARDs).

Red Blood Cell Count

Red blood cells carry oxygen from the lungs to the rest of the body. They contain hemoglobin, a protein that contains iron and gives blood its red color. Normal values for the RBC count range from 4.2 million to 5.9 million cmm (sometimes expressed simply as 4.2–5.9). Low RBC counts (also called anemia) can have multiple causes in a person with RA:

- RA itself
- A poor diet that includes low amounts of iron and protein
- Bleeding caused by aspirin or nonsteroidal anti-inflammatory drugs such as naproxen or ibuprofen

Platelet Count

Platelets (also called thrombocytes) are not actually blood cells, but rather are fragments of large blood-forming cells. These fragments are essential for normal blood clotting. The normal values for the PLT test vary between laboratories but are usually in the range of 150,000 to 400,000 cmm (sometimes expressed simply as 150–400). An increase in platelet count can be seen with RA, some blood diseases, and some cancers Low platelet counts may be seen in certain blood diseases and infections, and as the result of certain medications.

Your physician may check your CBC many times each year, depending on the activity of your disease, your symptoms, and the types of medications you are taking.

52. My doctor orders a complete blood count several times each year. Do I need to get this test so frequently?

A complete blood count (CBC) is an excellent screening test. It helps the doctor diagnose illnesses, monitor disease activity, and look out for medication side effects. How frequently a physician orders a CBC has a lot to do with your health history, your concurrent illnesses, the types of medications you are taking, and your present complaints.

The following examples describe how the CBC can be employed.

Case 1

A female patient with RA reports that lately she has been feeling weak, short of breath, and easily fatigued. This patient has a history of emphysema. A physical examination appears unchanged from her previous exam two months ago. A stool sample, however, is noted to contain traces of blood. It is not clear whether the fatigue and shortness of breath are related to the underlying RA, the emphysema, or some other medical problem. A CBC is ordered, and a low red blood cell count is noted; a diagnosis of anemia is made.

Later, the patient undergoes an endoscopy test that reveals the presence of gastric ulcers. The increased dose of ibuprofen taken by the patient is believed to be to blame for these ulcers. The patient's ulcers are treated, and her arthritis medication regimen is changed to avoid this complication. The patient receives a transfusion of two units of blood, and her symptoms of fatigue and shortness of breath improve dramatically.

Case 2

A patient limps into an emergency room at a local hospital. He complains of pain, swelling, and redness of his right knee for the past week. The pain appears to be getting worse, even though the patient has taken aspirin and used ice packs. The physician examines the knee, but is unsure if this is the first presentation of RA, a traumatic injury, or an infection. The doctor orders x-rays and a CBC, among other tests. The x-ray does not show any signs of fractures or dislocations. By contrast, the CBC demonstrates a markedly elevated white blood cell count, which suggests that the knee swelling is a result of an infection. The doctor uses a needle and syringe to aspirate a sample of the knee fluid. Under a microscope, the doctor can see many bacteria. A diagnosis of a knee joint infection is made—a condition called septic arthritis. After taking a course of antibiotics, the patient recovers fully.

Case 3

A 47-year-old woman complains of swelling and pain of her hands and wrists. She states that she has recently gone back to work as a secretary and is doing a lot of typing. She thinks that her pain could be from the typing. She has a history of RA, but states that this disease has only bothered her knees in the past. When the doctor examines the patient, he notes swelling of the wrists and knuckles of both of her hands. When the doctor takes a more detailed history, the patient states that she had noticed the swelling and mild stiffness before she returned to typing, and that both are worse when she gets up in the morning to go to work. The pain and stiffness seem to decrease by midmorning, especially if she takes aspirin or ibuprofen. She also mentions that she has experienced increasing fatigue: Working every day is a struggle, and she seems to tire more quickly than before.

The doctor orders a CBC, among other tests. The CBC indicates that the patient's white blood cell count is normal, but demonstrates a moderate decrease in the red blood cell count. This result suggests to the doctor that the patient does not have an acute infection, but rather has a moderate amount of anemia that is associated with active RA. The doctor diagnoses a worsening (flare) of the patient's RA. He institutes a more aggressive regimen of arthritis medication and prescribes iron supplements to help with her anemia. When he reassesses the patient after three months of treatment, both her joint pain and her fatigue have improved.

As you can tell from these examples, the CBC is useful in many clinical situations. It is a standard test that can help your doctor to both diagnose and monitor your disease.

53. What are antinuclear antibodies?

Antinuclear antibodies (ANA) are proteins found in the bloodstream of some people who have RA or other diseases. Doctors test for these antibodies to help make a diagnosis of RA and other autoimmune diseases such as systemic lupus erythematosus (SLE) and drug-induced lupus. An ANA test may also be positive in cases of scleroderma, Sjögren's syndrome, Raynaud's disease, juvenile chronic arthritis, antiphospholipid antibody syndrome, autoimmune hepatitis, and many other autoimmune and non-autoimmune diseases.

An antibody is part of the normal human immune system. The body uses such proteins to fight off infections caused by bacteria, viruses, and other infectious agents. Whereas the

Antinuclear antibody (ANA)

An unusual antibody that is directed against structures within the nucleus of the human cell. ANAs are found in patients whose immune systems are predisposed to cause inflammation against their own body tissues.

Testing for Rheumatoid Arthritis

typical antibodies bind to foreign material (e.g., bacterial cell walls), antinuclear antibodies act somewhat differently: They bind to structures within the center of the person's own cells. The center, or innermost core, of the cell is called the nucleus. It contains DNA along with other genetic material.

ANAs are found in patients whose immune systems may be predisposed to instigate inflammation against their own body tissues. Such antibodies, which are directed against a person's own tissues, are referred to as auto-antibodies. Thus ANAs are a sign of an autoimmune illness. When a person has an autoimmune disease, the immune system produces antibodies that attach to the body's own cells as though they were foreign substances, often causing them to be damaged or destroyed. Both RA and Crohn's disease (an inflammatory bowel disease) are examples of autoimmune diseases. A thorough medical history, physical examination, and other tests besides an ANA test are needed to confirm the diagnosis of a suspected autoimmune disease.

The ANA test is performed using a small sample of blood usually taken from your arm. In traditional laboratory ANA testing, your blood serum is placed in a container with specially grown human cells. If your blood contains antibodies to the tissues in a human cell, they will stick to the cells in the container and can be detected using certain chemicals and a special microscope. Newer, more rapid laboratory techniques are also commonly used to confirm the presence of ANAs. Regardless of which technique is used, the laboratory measures two characteristics of the ANA in your blood: the amount of antibody and the pattern (what the antibody sticks to in the cell).

The amount of antibody is measured by a titer, which indicates how many times the technician could dilute the patient's blood and still detect the presence of ANAs. A titer of 1 to 80 (1:80) means that antibodies could be last detected when 1 part of the blood sample was diluted by 80 parts of another liquid (usually a dilute salt solution). A larger second number indicates that the antibodies are present in greater concentration. For example, a titer of 1:320 indicates a higher concentration of antibodies in the blood than a titer of 1:80, because it took 320 dilutions to get to an undetectable amount of ANA in the former sample versus 80 dilutions in the latter sample. Given that each dilution involves doubling the amount of test fluid, it is not surprising that titers increase rapidly. In fact, the difference between titers of 1:160 and 1:320 is only a single dilution, so it doesn't necessarily represent a major difference in disease activity. Such variability is very common, especially if more than one laboratory is involved in processing the samples.

The amount of ANA in your bloodstream will inevitably go up and down during the course of the disease. For this reason, physicians don't consider the ANA titers to be an accurate reflection of disease activity. A titer of 1:80 or lower is usually considered to be a negative test result.

When looking for the ANA pattern, the technician examines a specially prepared slide under a microscope. ANAs can present as four different "patterns" depending on where the antibodies adhere to the cell nucleus: homogeneous (diffuse), speckled, nucleolar, and peripheral (rim). While these patterns are not specific to any one illness, certain illnesses are more frequently associated with one pattern or another. Thus the patterns can sometimes give the doctor further clues about the types of illnesses to look for when evaluating a patient. For example, the nucleolar pattern is more commonly encountered in scleroderma, the rim (peripheral) pattern is the most specific pattern for lupus, and the homogeneous (diffuse) pattern is the most common pattern seen overall. The speckled pattern is seen in many conditions and in persons who have no autoimmune disease at all.

Testing for Rheumatoid Arthritis

No one test can "prove" that a person has RA. Instead, RA is diagnosed only after your doctor has performed a full history and physical exam and administered a few tests, such as the antinuclear antibody test.

54. Does a positive antinuclear antibody test mean that I have rheumatoid arthritis?

No one test can "prove" that a person has RA, or any other autoimmune disease for that matter. Instead, RA is diagnosed only after your doctor has performed a full history and physical exam and administered a few tests, such as the antinuclear antibody (ANA) test. You should consider the following facts when thinking about your ANA test results.

First, ANAs can be "normal." These auto-antibodies are found in approximately 5% of the normal (i.e., without RA) population, usually in low titers (low levels). These persons usually experience no joint symptoms and have no disease. ANA titers less than 1:80 are less likely to be significant, and ANA titers less than or equal to 1:40 are considered negative. Even higher titers are often insignificant in persons who are more than 60 years of age.

Second, certain medications may lead to elevated ANA titers. Before taking this test, you should inform your doctor if you are taking any of the following medications, as they can interfere with the accuracy of the test:

- Hydralazine (Apresoline), procainamide (Procan, Pronestyl, Promine), and certain anticonvulsants (Dilantin, Mysoline)
- Antibiotics (isoniazid, penicillin, tetracycline), birth control pills, lithium, and some diuretics, such as chlorthalidone (Hygroton)
- Heart or blood pressure medications, such as acebutolol (Sectral), captopril (Capoten), atenolol (Tenormin), metoprolol (Lopressor), lovastatin (Mevacor), and quinidine
- Steroids, which may cause a false-negative result

Third, elevated ANA titers may be found in patients with the following non-arthritic diseases:

- Infections (viral or bacterial)
- Lung diseases (primary pulmonary fibrosis, pulmonary hypertension)
- Gastrointestinal diseases (ulcerative colitis, Crohn's disease, primary biliary cirrhosis, alcoholic liver disease)
- Hormonal diseases (Hashimoto's autoimmune thyroiditis, Graves' disease)
- Blood diseases (idiopathic thrombocytopenic purpura, hemolytic anemia)
- Cancers (melanoma, breast, lung, kidney, ovarian, and others)
- Skin diseases (psoriasis, pemphigus)

Your doctor should ask you about any other illnesses you have during your medical history. If reading this list reminds you of a disease you've had in the past, let your doctor know.

Your physician will be aware of the limitations of the ANA test. For instance, your physician knows that a positive ANA test may or may not be significant in a given individual, but merely helps to support a diagnosis that is based on your clinical history and physical examination. A positive ANA test helps to support a diagnosis of RA *if* you have physical signs and symptoms of the disease. The ANA is highly sensitive but nonspecific, however, so it produces a high number of false-positive results.

In the past, before the limitations of ANA tests were well understood, these tests were ordered frequently but not always appropriately. Unfortunately, a positive ANA test in an otherwise healthy person often began a time-consuming and expensive search for a nonexistent autoimmune disease, causing a lot of needless worry and anxiety on the part of the patient. Today, an ANA test is rarely ordered unless your physician has a strong suspicion that you are suffering from an autoimmune disease, such as RA.

Testing for Rheumatoid Arthritis

Citrulline antibody

An antibody directed against an unusual amino acid called citrulline. Citrulline is not normally present in peptides or proteins in the body. The presence of high amounts of the citrulline antibody in the bloodstream suggests that the person is suffering from rheumatoid arthritis.

55. What is the citrulline antibody test?

A newer blood test used to help diagnose RA is the **citrulline antibody** test, more formally known as the cyclic citrullinated peptide (CCP) antibody test. It may also be referred to as anti-citrulline antibody, anti-cyclic citrullinated peptide antibody (anti-CCP), or cyclic citrullinated peptide antibody IgG (CCP IgG).

Like rheumatoid factor (RF), CCP is an antibody that is produced in a person who has an autoimmune disease. This antibody is directed against an unusual amino acid called citrulline. Citrulline is formed when amino groups are removed from arginine, a natural amino acid. Medical research suggests that in the joints of patients with RA, proteins may be changed to citrulline through some unknown process. The body's immune system treats this protein as foreign material and creates antibodies to it—that is, anti-CCP antibodies. These antibodies begin to attack the joints, in an action that some scientists believe causes the inflammation of the rheumatoid joint. Measuring the citrulline antibody provides the basis for a screening test for RA. Citrulline antibodies are measured with a blood test that is analyzed in a laboratory.

Compared with test for RF, the test for citrulline antibodies is both more sensitive and more specific for RA. A more sensitive test means that a higher percentage of people with RA will have a positive CCP test, as compared with the RF test. A more specific test means that when a person has a positive CCP result, he or she is more likely to truly have RA, as compared with having a positive RF test.

In one study, CCP antibodies were found in 76% of patients with confirmed RA, but a positive RF test was obtained in only 60% of the same patients. When patients had RA and tested positive for RF, the rate of positive CCP antibody tests increased to 90%. In patients with confirmed RA whose RF tests were negative, the CCP antibody test was positive in only

40%. In healthy volunteers, a CCP antibody test was positive in only 1% of patients—a better performance than the test for RF, which was positive in as many as 10% of healthy volunteers. Therefore, a positive CCP test is more likely to mean a true diagnosis of RA than a positive RF test. Further, the CCP test will give fewer false-positive results when compared to a RF test (1% versus 10%, respectively.)

The CCP antibody also appears earlier in the course of RA than RF, so the CCP test can be used to detect early-stage RA disease. In one study, this test was positive in patients with RA who had joint symptoms for only three to six months. Another study suggested that CCP antibodies may predate the onset of arthritis symptoms by several years in some patients. For all these reasons, it may be a good idea for people with positive CCP blood tests to visit their doctor on a regular basis, even if they have not been officially diagnosed with RA.

56. When should my doctor order a citrulline antibody test?

Testing positive for the CCP antibody test does not automatically mean that you have RA. A CCP test can be positive in other rheumatic diseases, such as systemic lupus erythematosus, Sjögren's syndrome, scleroderma, and cryoglobulinemia, as well as in some infectious diseases. In addition, 1% of healthy people will have positive CCP tests.

Some studies have indicated that patients with RA who have CCP antibodies early in the course of their disease tend to develop RA that is more destructive to the joints. Other investigators have confirmed this relationship and have suggested that the CCP test is superior to the RF test in predicting the severity of RA. The use of this test may, therefore, help your physician to decide whether you should undergo a more aggressive (and riskier) treatment course at an earlier stage of the disease.

Testing positive for the CCP antibody test does not automatically mean that you have RA.

Testing for Rheumatoid Arthritis

Based on these and other studies, physicians recommend that a CCP antibody test should be ordered in the following situations:

- When you have signs and symptoms of RA, but your test for RF is negative or equivocal.
- When you are at high risk for having RA based on your physical exam and other diagnostic tests, and your doctor wants to increase the accuracy of the diagnosis.
- When you have no signs or symptoms of RA, but a RF test is positive, and your doctor wants to eliminate the chance that you may have early-stage RA without joint symptoms.
- When you have been positively diagnosed with RA and your physician wants to monitor your disease activity.
- When you have been positively diagnosed with RA and your physician wants to evaluate your prognosis and make decisions about future treatment. That is, this test is used when your doctor suspects that you will have a more destructive form of RA and would like to use the CCP test results to help decide whether more aggressive therapy is warranted.

57. What is C-reactive protein?

C-reactive protein (CRP) is found in the bloodstream of people who have an inflammatory condition such as RA. This protein is made in the liver and its production increases when inflammation is present in the body (though it is not the only protein that is produced when inflammation occurs). CRP plays an important role in the immune system, helping other proteins to destroy foreign material such as bacteria, viruses, and fungi. Physicians test for it because CRP is reasonably specific for inflammation and the test is easy to perform.

A higher level of CRP in the blood indicates a higher level of disease activity. In this sense, the CRP is similar to the erythrocyte sedimentation rate (ESR, also called the "sed rate").

Like the sed rate, the CRP level is an indicator of inflammation, but it is not a specific test for RA. A high level of CRP does not mean a person has RA, and some people with active RA have a low level of CRP—or even no CRP at all. The reason for this aberration is not known. Thus a low CRP level does not always mean that inflammation is not present.

A normal, healthy person should not have a CRP level. Physicians consider a CRP level higher than 1 mg/dL to be elevated. For most infections and significant inflammatory diseases, CRP levels in excess of 10 mg/dL are the norm.

A positive CRP test may be an indicator of several conditions, including RA, rheumatic fever, cancer, tuberculosis, pneumonia, heart attack, bone, joint and skin infections, and systemic lupus erythematosus. An elevated CRP level also can be detected during the last half of a normal pregnancy or in women who are taking oral contraceptives.

Although the sed rate and the CRP level both tend to increase with increased inflammation, sometimes one measure will be raised while the other is normal. This discrepancy can occur because CRP levels rise more rapidly and disappear more quickly than changes in the sed rate. As a result, your CRP level may fall to normal if you have been treated successfully, such as for a flare of arthritis, but your ESR may still be abnormal for a while longer. In light of these differences, doctors often order both the sed rate and CRP tests to make sure they can detect changes in your disease process. The CRP is repeated regularly to monitor the level of your inflammation and your response to medication, because CRP levels drop as inflammation subsides.

The "normal" range for the CRP level may change depending on which laboratory is analyzing your blood sample. If your CRP level is tested repeatedly at the same lab, increases and decreases in this level may be meaningful. Conversely, if

Testing for Rheumatoid Arthritis

your blood is tested in different laboratories that use different "normal ranges," then changes in the CRP level must be judged with caution.

A CRP level is measured from a small sample of blood that is drawn from a vein, usually from the inside of your elbow or the back of your hand. No special preparation or fasting is required before the blood is drawn.

58. Why does my doctor need to do an x-ray?

When a physician is evaluating a person with joint pain and swelling, he or she may use x-rays to determine whether the arthritis has caused damage to the bones of the joint. Radiographs, as x-rays are sometimes called, are especially important if the doctor suspects RA. He or she will often order that x-rays be taken of any swollen joints. Although x-rays cannot confirm the presence of RA, they can be a useful tool for distinguishing between RA, osteoarthritis, and other conditions. Additionally, x-rays establish a baseline for comparison. As the disease progresses, they can be used to monitor changes in the bones over time. Early in the course of the disease, the bone changes associated with RA do not always appear on x-rays because bone damage is not yet visible. In general, x-rays are more useful later in the disease, when bones may be affected more dramatically.

Early in the course of the disease, the bone changes associated with RA do not always appear on x-rays. In general, x-rays are more useful later in the disease, when bones may be affected more dramatically.

Often, as part of a person's initial evaluation with a rheumatologist, chest x-rays are ordered in addition to x-rays of any swollen joints. Chest x-rays are performed to evaluate the lung for diseases that are sometimes associated with arthritis (see Question 18).

X-rays are usually performed in a special hospital department (Radiology) by a radiologic technician or a radiographer, who will tell you which part of your body is to be imaged. These technicians are highly skilled. They must have college degrees, receive additional training in their field, and pass a state licensing examination before they can take x-rays. The training for a radiologic technician is different from that of a radiologist; the latter professional is a physician who is trained to interpret x-ray images.

To make the image, x-rays are passed through your body and captured on special film. This x-ray film is then developed and examined. Standard x-rays are particularly good at showing abnormalities of the bone. Unfortunately, because they rarely show problems in soft tissues, x-rays cannot show early signs of arthritis very well. Despite this drawback, examination of x-rays can help the doctor to diagnose arthritis by highlighting damaged areas on the bone.

The way bones appear on x-rays can vary in normal people and changes occur with age. For example, age-related abnormalities are frequently seen on x-rays of the spine, even in people without pain. Many people may have normal-looking x-rays despite suffering severe pain from inflammation in or around the joints. In addition, x-rays can show apparent damage or abnormalities that may not be the cause of the pain, swelling, or stiffness. For these reasons, your doctor will not rely on x-rays alone to make the diagnosis of RA, but will interpret the images alongside findings from the physical examination or other tests.

Other Imaging Methods

In addition to the standard x-ray of the joint or bone, other ways of imaging the body are used to identify signs of RA.

In arthrography, dye is injected into the joint to allow it to show up in more detail when x-rayed. Occasionally, dye may be injected into a blood vessel to assess the circulation under x-ray (this is called an arteriogram or venogram).

Computerized tomography (CT) uses x-rays that record images of sections or "slices" of the body. These multiple images

Testing for Rheumatoid Arthritis

are then processed by a computer to produce cross-sectional pictures of the body part. CT scans can give detailed pictures of the skeleton, but will also show other types of tissue, such as the muscles, which cannot be seen on an ordinary x-ray.

An isotope is a chemical that gives off a type of radioactivity called gamma rays. In an isotope bone scan, a very small amount of the isotope is injected into the blood and is taken up by the bones. The gamma rays are then detected by a special camera, and this information is sent to a computer, which combines the data to build a picture showing which areas of the bone are inflamed. The dose of radiation delivered with this imaging technique is very small and will quickly be excreted from the body in the urine.

Magnetic resonance imaging (MRI)

A diagnostic technique in which radio waves generated in a strong magnetic field are used to provide information about the hydrogen atoms in different tissues within the body. A computer then uses this information to produce images of the tissues in many different planes.

Magnetic resonance imaging (MRI) uses high-frequency radio waves in a strong magnetic field to produce highly detailed pictures of the body. The radio waves interact with the water molecules in the body's tissues, and the signals that come back are processed by a computer to build up pictures of the inside of the body. An MRI scan produces pictures of the soft tissues—particularly cartilage, tendons, and nerves—that cannot be detected by x-rays. This technique is often used to detect early or minor abnormalities in these soft tissues; it can also detect signs of inflammation. MRI scans are particularly useful for the spine, the shoulder, and the knee. They can show numerous differences between individuals, many of which are completely normal, so it is important that the results be interpreted by the doctor who has ordered the imaging investigation.

PART SEVEN

Nonpharmaceutical Therapies for Rheumatoid Arthritis: When Pills Are Not Enough

What can I do to improve my energy level?

How do I reduce the stress on my joints?

Can surgery improve the symptoms
of rheumatoid arthritis?

More ...

59. What can I do to improve my energy level?

Fatigue is a common symptom of RA and can be a difficult problem to manage. To improve fatigue, it is important to find out *why* you are fatigued. Your doctor can help by taking a good medical history, including asking about the duration and quality of your sleep, the amount of pain you are having, the amount of joint swelling and stiffness you are experiencing, and any signs of stomach ulcers or blood loss that might cause anemia. The physical exam should not only concentrate on your joints, but also include checks for other physical problems that could make you more fatigued, such as heart, lung, or thyroid disease.

You should review each of the common causes of fatigue and work with your physician to treat them.

The Inflammatory Process Itself

The amount of inflammation your body is experiencing will have an effect on your energy level. People with RA often state that their level of fatigue increases with the amount of joint pain and tenderness. Treatment of the inflammation reduces fatigue. Therefore, compliance with your medication is an important way to improve fatigue. You should inform your doctor about any disease flares. He or she may suggest a temporary increase in the dose of one medication or the temporary addition of another medication to relieve the increased inflammation.

Chronic Pain

Treating your pain is important, because chronic pain can cause a lack of sleep or nonrefreshing sleep, increased fatigue, and depression. Discuss your level of pain with your physician. Localized pain may be treated with hot packs, massages, or steroid injections into inflamed joints. More diffuse pain can be treated with nonsteroidal pain relievers or stronger medications, including morphine and its derivatives. If your pain is not under control despite the best efforts of your rheumatologist, he or she may suggest that you consult with a pain specialist.

In some cases, some painful joints may improve dramatically after surgery. For this reason, a consultation with an orthopedic surgeon is appropriate in some cases of chronic pain.

Poor Sleep Quality

Tell your doctor if you're not sleeping well, because poor sleep quality is one measure of the effectiveness of your RA treatment regimen. Discuss with your physician what kind of problem is keeping you from getting a full night's sleep. Is it pain? Is it anxiety? Is it an inability to get out of bed to go to the bathroom? Each of these issues can be treated and can improve the quality of your sleep.

Depression

Signs of depression include lack of motivation, tearfulness, and inability to enjoy the things that once brought you pleasure. Your physician can often diagnose depression quickly in his or her office by asking a set of standardized questions. Treatment of depression may include psychological counseling, medication, or both. A psychologist, for example, may be able to help you identify coping mechanisms that will allow you to deal with your disease more effectively. In addition, many new antidepressant medications that are highly effective and have few side effects are available.

Anemia

Anemia can be diagnosed with a simple blood test. If anemia (that is, a low red blood cell count) is found, your physician will have to identify its cause. This investigation may involve a test of your stool for signs of blood loss indicating internal bleeding from the stomach or intestines. You should report abdominal pain and any changes in the color of your stool, as they may be signs of stomach ulcers. The medications used to treat the inflammation of your RA can improve or eliminate the anemia of chronic disease.

Lack of Exercise

Medical research has consistently demonstrated the benefits of exercise for people with RA. Exercise improves the functioning of the heart, lungs, muscles, and joints. It also reduces your risk for coronary artery disease, osteoporosis, and overweight and obesity. Patients who participate in regular exercise programs typically report that they begin to sleep better and that their pain and fatigue levels decrease.

If you find it difficult to start an exercise regimen, consult with a physical therapist or rehabilitation specialist. He or she can design an exercise program that's tailored to your age and condition.

All people with RA will suffer from fatigue from time to time. If your fatigue is debilitating or prolonged, discuss it with your doctor and get it treated.

All people with RA will suffer from fatigue from time to time. If your fatigue is debilitating or prolonged, discuss it with your doctor and get it treated.

60. How do I reduce the stress on my joints?

Mechanical stress on inflamed joints can worsen the pain and increase the damage that arthritis causes. While medication can help to decrease the inflammation associated with RA, reducing the stress on your joints can help both to reduce pain and to prevent disability.

The majority of joint stress is caused by increased body weight and inappropriate exercise. Obesity, for example, places tremendous stress on the weight-bearing joints in the low back, hips, knees, ankles, and feet—all of which are commonly inflamed by RA. If you suffer from RA, you should set a goal to achieve and maintain an ideal body weight. Meeting this target can reduce your risk of heart attack, stroke, and diabetes as well as improve your joint pain and prevent disability.

Getting enough rest is another important feature of RA management. When your joints are actively inflamed, you should avoid engaging in vigorous activity. Activity in this setting, for example, can intensify joint inflammation or cause traumatic injury to structures weakened by inflammation.

While rest is very important, especially when acute joint inflammation occurs, careful exercise is also encouraged for patients with RA. Exercise is necessary to prevent wasting of the muscles and improve cardiovascular health. Thus performing modest amounts of exercise when joints are not inflamed is recommended. Some people are able to get safe exercise even during a flare of their arthritis. For example, they can exercise their arms and shoulders when their knees are inflamed or walk more when their wrists and hands hurt.

Some mechanical aids are effective in reducing joint stress:

- *Splints.* Splinting of acutely inflamed joints, particularly at night, reduces pain and joint stress. Splinting has a modest anti-inflammatory effect, but may increase stiffness.
- *Walking Aids.* Employing a cane or a walker can be an effective means of reducing stress on the hip, knee, and ankle joints. Wheelchairs and motorized mobility devices may also be appropriate, even for ambulatory patients, during flares of arthritis in their lower extremities.
- *Grasping Aids.* Using pliers to open bottles, twist caps, or grab the tops of pots or cooking utensils can reduce stress in your hands and wrists. Long-handled "pickups" such as those used by gardeners or cleanup crews, can decrease stress on your hands as well as your back and knees. The long handle means that you do not have to bend down to pick up things. Many tools and utensils are now sold with "built-up" foam handles that make them easier to grip and manipulate.

Nonpharmaceutical Therapies for Rheumatoid Arthritis: When Pills Are Not Enough

- *Remote-Control Devices.* Using remote-control devices can decrease the amount of walking you must do in your home. The remote control for the television is common enough, but remote controls can also be used to adjust the room's thermostat, open front doors, turn on and off lights, and access security systems. Using a cordless telephone or cell phone may also reduce the number of times you have to run to answer the phone.

Discuss these and other aids and devices with your rheumatologist, physical therapist, or occupational therapist. Consultations with a physical therapist and an occupational therapist are recommended for everyone early in the course of RA. These specialists can advise you on exercise and mechanical aids, suggesting which ones are most helpful and letting you know where to purchase them.

61. Can surgery improve the symptoms of rheumatoid arthritis?

Rheumatoid arthritis is an inflammatory process that affects the synovium, and its symptoms generally respond to the various anti-inflammatory medications that constitute the armamentarium of the rheumatologist. Sometimes, however, RA-induced changes to the structural or mechanical alignment of a joint may cause pain, disfigurement, or loss of joint function. In these cases, the pain, function, and appearance of the joint may be improved by surgery. Several types of surgery are available to patients with severe joint damage, including total or partial joint replacement, tendon reconstruction, and synovectomy.

Arthroplasty

Implantation of a mechanical joint to replace a diseased or damaged joint; also called total joint replacement surgery.

Joint Replacement

Total joint replacement, also known as joint **arthroplasty,** involves replacing the damaged natural joint with an artificial joint. Joint replacements are the most commonly performed surgery for RA and are highly successful in relieving pain, improving joint appearance, and preserving joint function. They are most commonly applied to the knee (**total knee replacement**), hip (**total hip replacement**), shoulder, and knuckles of the hands. The new joint, called a prosthesis, is made of metal alloys, plastics, and sometimes ceramic. Such joints are highly durable and sometimes last more than 20 years. Unfortunately, artificial joints can wear out with excessive use, so they may not be the best option for younger people.

Complications can occasionally arise following joint replacement surgery if the artificial joint does not attach well, the bones are damaged, or the joint becomes infected or loosened through wear or inflammation. Nevertheless, most artificial joints work well, and many people experience significant pain relief from them.

Tendon Reconstruction

Tendons are strong, fibrous tissues that attach muscles to bones. The inflammatory process of RA can damage and even rupture tendons, particularly the extensor tendons of the hand or wrist. If that happens, the affected finger cannot be fully extended unless surgical repair of the tendon is undertaken. Tendon reconstruction repairs the damaged tendon by attaching an intact tendon to it. This procedure can restore joint function, particularly if it is done early, before the tendon becomes completely ruptured.

Synovectomy

Synovectomy is a procedure to remove the joint lining (synovium) that has been damaged by RA. In two medical studies that followed the long-term results of synovectomy in patients with RA, researchers found that most patients continued to experience improved joint function for as long as eight or nine years. Unfortunately, some patients' joints continued to deteriorate after surgery owing to the regrowth of the synovium.

The timing of synovectomy is important, because this surgery is more effective in improving function if it is performed

Total knee replacement

A surgical procedure in which damaged parts of the knee joint are replaced with artificial parts, which are usually made of plastic and steel.

Total hip replacement

A type of surgery in which the diseased ball and socket of the hip joint are completely removed and replaced with artificial materials. Also called a hip arthroplasty.

Synovectomy

Removal of the synovial membrane of a joint.

before significant bone and cartilage destruction occurs. Function is also improved when synovectomy is done in combination with tendon reconstruction.

Other Surgical Procedures

Other operations performed in patients with RA include removal of tissue that presses on nerves, such as the nerve entrapments that occur with carpal tunnel syndrome; arthroscopic procedures to the knee and hip; and skin surgery to remove a symptomatic rheumatoid nodule.

Issues to Consider Before Surgery

Surgery is not appropriate for all people who have RA.

Surgery is not appropriate for all people who have RA. As with any treatment, there are risks to consider. Your primary care physician, rheumatologist, and orthopedist should help you to understand the risks and benefits of having the surgical procedure as well as the risks and benefits of not having surgery. Be sure to discuss the following issues with your physician before you make your decision:

- The need for joint replacement
- The likely outcome of the surgery
- The cost of the surgery
- Insurance reimbursement
- Your motivation and goals
- Your ability to undergo rehabilitation (this is sometimes more difficult than the surgery itself)
- Lost work and lost wages associated with rehabilitation
- Your general medical status
- Surgical- and anesthesia-related risks
- The functional life of the joint prosthesis and the possible need for its replacement (Replacement of the replacement is sometimes called a "revision" procedure.)

After a thorough discussion of these issues, you and your doctor can decide whether surgery is right for you.

62. I've heard that I can have my blood "filtered" to treat my rheumatoid arthritis. Is that possible?

Yes, there is a device that treats RA by "filtering" the blood—the so-called extracorporeal immunoadsorption protein A column. While its name sounds complex, the device's function is based on a simple theory: Antibodies have a tendency to stick to certain proteins, so this blood-filtering technique exploits that tendency. In the United States, this filtering device is sold under the name Prosorba Column.

The filtering device is a plastic cylinder that measures three by six inches, or approximately the size of a coffee mug. The cylinder contains a sand-like substance called silica that is coated with a special material called Protein A. Protein A has the unique property of being able to stick to the antibodies in the blood of patients with RA, some of which actually attack the body's own tissues (leading to RA). The patient's blood is circulated from a needle in the vein of one arm, through this filter, and then to a needle in a vein of the patient's other arm. As the blood flows through the filter, the antibodies that cause RA stick to the protein in the column and are removed from the blood. After this treatment, the patient has significantly less antibodies in his or her bloodstream.

This procedure is usually performed once a week for 12 weeks in an outpatient setting. Each treatment takes between one and two hours. Many patients experience significant relief in arthritis symptoms that can last for six to eight months.

Many patients breeze through this blood-filtering procedure with little or no discomfort. Others have experienced adverse reactions, including joint pain, fatigue, joint swelling, low blood pressure, nausea, chest pain, shortness of breath, and allergic reactions. While these reactions are not common, the doctor must watch out for them.

Treatment with the Prosorba Column is indicated for patients who have long-standing RA that is either moderate or severe. Additionally, these patients must have failed to respond to conventional drug therapy or be intolerant to those medications. By contrast, patients with the following conditions should not undergo this kind of blood-filtering therapy:

Enzyme

Any protein that regulates chemical changes in other substances.

- Individuals who are receiving angiotensin-converting **enzyme** (ACE) inhibitor medications
- Individuals who have serious heart or lung problems
- Individuals who cannot tolerate a similar procedure called apheresis
- Individuals who have demonstrated a prior allergy or hypersensitivity to this therapy
- Individuals who have a tendency to form blood clots (hypercoagulability)

The long-term safety and effectiveness of this therapy is unknown, but is currently being studied.

63. Is alternative or complementary medicine helpful for rheumatoid arthritis?

Alternative medicine and *complementary medicine* are terms that are often used interchangeably. We will follow this practice in this text.

Alternative medicine comprises a mixed group of practices that target hygiene, diagnosis, and treatment of many diseases. The theoretical bases of alternative medicine diverge from those of modern scientific medicine and are not generally accepted by modern physicians. Alternative medicine has failed to gain widespread acceptance because these practices currently lack a plausible scientific basis. Furthermore, few studies have demonstrated their safety and efficacy.

Alternative medicine may emerge from any of the following sources:

- Religious sources
- Cultural beliefs
- Supernatural, magical, or cultist practices
- Naive, illogical, or false understandings of anatomy, physiology, pathology, or pharmacology
- Fraud and exploitation of the sick and hopeless

Any treatment that is outside the traditional medicine or practice of your primary health system can be considered alternative medicine. Of course, a treatment that is considered to be "alternative" in one culture may be deemed "traditional" in another culture. For example, acupuncture is a system of treatment that has been practiced in China for more than 5000 years, yet is considered an alternative medicine in the United States.

Practitioners of Western (allopathic) medicine are closely monitored and regulated in the United States, and must undergo rigorous training and testing as well as licensing by state and federal authorities. The facilities of modern practitioners, such as hospitals, surgical centers, and dialysis units, are subject to similar scrutiny and licensing requirements. By contrast, complementary medicine practitioners and their therapies are rarely—if ever—subject to this level of testing and regulatory oversight in the United States. Therefore, patients who seek out these therapies cannot be confident in the abilities of the practitioners to safely practice their remedies.

The greatest risk involved with using complementary medicine is the risk of missing a necessary or possibly life-saving diagnosis or treatment from a practitioner of conventional medicine. In RA, early treatment with one of the newer medications can significantly inhibit joint destruction. Using an alternative medicine that lacks the same properties could lead to irreversible joint damage and disability.

Other problems associated with complementary therapies include the potential for dangerous interactions with conventional

In RA, early treatment with one of the newer medications can significantly inhibit joint destruction. Using an alternative medicine that lacks the same properties could lead to irreversible joint damage and disability.

therapies. Many complementary therapies also lack evidence of effectiveness (most have not been subjected to rigorous clinical trials). Also, many complementary therapies may not be covered by health insurance.

The growing consumer interest in alternative medicine has expanded the market for a wide range of products, from acupuncture to the flood of dietary supplements that are now on the market. Supplements are popular, but questions remain about the safety of some of these products. In 1994, the U.S. Congress decided that dietary supplements should be regulated as if they were foods. In other words, these products are assumed to be safe unless the Food and Drug Administration (FDA) can demonstrate that they pose a significant risk to consumers. Manufacturers are not legally required to provide specific information about supplements' safety and effectiveness before marketing their products. Furthermore, some supplements may interfere with the effectiveness of your other RA medications. For all these reasons, you should use caution when taking supplements and do so only after discussing these products with your treating physician.

The following are some alternative medicine treatments you may want to discuss with your physician.

Acupuncture

Acupuncture is commonly used by patients with chronic painful musculoskeletal disorders. There are, however, few well-designed studies that demonstrate its efficacy.

Glucosamine and Chondroitin Sulfate

Glucosamine and **chondroitin sulfate** are natural substances found in and around the cells of cartilage. Glucosamine is an amino sugar that the body produces and distributes in cartilage and other connective tissue. Chondroitin sulfate is a complex carbohydrate that helps cartilage retain water. In the United States, glucosamine and chondroitin sulfate are

Glucosamine

An amino sugar produced by the body that is found in cartilage. Glucosamine is a popular dietary supplement and is thought to improve the joints symptoms of osteoarthritis.

Chondroitin sulfate

A sugar-based material that is present in cartilage. Chondroitin is a popular dietary supplement that is thought to improve the joint symptoms of osteoarthritis.

sold as dietary supplements; hence, they are regulated as foods rather than drugs. Recent medical trials have shown that glucosamine and chondroitin sulfate are more effective than placebo in relieving pain from osteoarthritis of the knee. As yet, however, similar studies demonstrating these supplements' effectiveness in relieving pain in patients with RA have not been performed. Before trying glucosamine or chondroitin sulfate, discuss this choice with your doctor and ask how it would fit in with your current treatment program.

Hydrotherapy

Hydrotherapy is the use of water in the treatment of disease. Hydrothermal therapy also exploits temperature-related effects, as in hot baths, saunas, and wraps. Hydrotherapy may make patients feel better by taking the weight off of painful joints, allowing them to participate in exercise classes and helping them to relax afterward. It has not been shown to affect the course of RA or to be able to replace drug therapy.

Herbs

Ginseng is a root that has been used to treat patients with a variety of illnesses for the last 2000 years, particularly in Asian cultures. To date, research results on Asian ginseng are not conclusive enough to prove the many health claims associated with the herb. Only a handful of large clinical trials on Asian ginseng have been conducted to date. Most studies have been small or have had flaws in design and reporting. Some claims for health benefits have been based only on studies conducted in animals.

Antioxidants, such as vitamin C and E, may help reduce the oxidative damage that occurs during flare ups of RA. As yet, no studies have demonstrated that the use of antioxidants results in an improvement in RA symptoms.

Fatty acids are the building materials of fats. Although most fatty acids can be produced in your body, the essential fatty acids need to be part of your diet, because your body cannot manufacture them. There are two essential fatty acids, called alpha linolenic acid and linoleic acid. Alpha linolenic acid (also known as omega-3 fatty acid) is found in flax seed, walnuts, and canola oil. Linoleic acid (also known as omega-6 fatty acid) is found in soy, sunflower seeds, corn oil, and most nuts. Some medical studies suggest that gamma-linolenic acid, which is found in evening primrose oil, can produce a subjective improvement in symptoms and allow some patients to reduce or stop treatment with nonsteroidal anti-inflammatory drugs (NSAIDs). There is, however, no evidence that they act as disease-modifying agents.

Aromatherapy is a treatment wherein the body and especially the face are massaged with preparations of fragrant essential oils. These oils are extracted from herbs, flowers, and fruits. Aromatherapy may be of some benefit in patients with RA, but more convincing research is needed to prove their efficacy.

Biofeedback

Biofeedback has been used to reduce stress and relieve anxiety in many studies. Research regarding its use in RA is lacking.

Yoga

For thousands of years, people have used yoga to build flexibility, strength, improve concentration, relieve stress, and increase energy. Medical studies have demonstrated that yoga can improve strength and flexibility in patients with RA, and yoga exercises have been created especially for these patients. A guide to these exercises, called *The Remain Active with RA Yoga Guide,* is offered for free at www.RAacademy.com and can be accessed after you register as a visitor to the site.

Exercise

Many people with RA may benefit from low-impact exercises. These exercises help improve overall health and fitness without further damaging or hurting the joints. Exercise has repeatedly been shown to improve quality of life, endurance, and lung function in patients with RA.

Massage

Patients with RA may complain of muscle pain as well as joint pain. Muscle pain can be the result of either muscle tension associated with joint pain or an abnormal gait produced by a swollen knee or ankle. Massaging sore muscles can help them to relax; indeed, many people feel better after a massage. Massage therapy has not been shown to alter the course of RA or to reduce inflammation in the joints.

Therapeutic Bracelets

The marketers of several brands of therapeutic bracelets have made unsubstantiated claims regarding their use in the treatment of arthritis. These manufacturers have claimed that the unique properties of the bracelet—for example, its composition, ionization, and electrical or magnetic charge—have curative effects for arthritis sufferers. This treatment rationale is complete nonsense. Not surprisingly, little or no clinical testing has been performed in an attempt to substantiate these claims. The FDA and the Federal Trade Commission (FTC) have sued several of these manufacturers for making false claims and for failing to honor advertised "money back" guarantees.

Homeopathic Remedies

Homeopaths use remedies that come from many different sources. Most are derived from plants, but minerals and metals may also be used in these therapies. After the initial preparation of the raw materials, these components are put into solutions of water or alcohol and turned into "remedies." The liquid is then used as a treatment or soaked into tablets or granules for convenience. No controlled clinical studies have shown that these remedies are any more effective than taking sugar pills.

With any treatment, it is always best to get as much information as possible; this is especially true regarding unregulated complementary therapies. After you've gathered all the necessary information regarding the benefits and risks of a treatment, you can then make an informed decision in consultation with your doctor.

64. Should I modify my home?

Given that RA is a disease that can affect mobility and strength, home modifications can make your life much easier. Some home modifications are simpler to make than others. For example, moving from a multilevel home to a single-level home or apartment is a big change, but even small accommodations can make a big difference.

Home modifications can make your life much easier. Even small accommodations can make a big difference.

Arthritis of the hips or knees makes getting up and down from a low seat much more difficult and painful than it is for people without arthritis. Avoiding low chairs is essential. Lift chairs can be helpful, but they are expensive, and many insurance programs require your doctor to provide documentation before they will pay for these devices.

An elevated commode seat is an inexpensive home improvement that will make getting up and down from the toilet easier. Grab bars for the commode and bathtub or shower are also important for accessibility and safety. If getting up and down in the bathtub is difficult, a metal shower stool is another inexpensive device that will make life easier.

Removing doorway thresholds is very helpful for people who use wheelchairs or scooters. If there are stairs at the front door or the house has a front stoop, then a ramp will be needed. Wide doorways and hallways are necessary to ensure accessibility to all rooms of the house.

Lowering the kitchen counters to the level of the wheelchair may also be required. Conversely, platforms for elevating appliances such as dishwashers or washing machines can save you from a lot of bending over. Special door handles that are easier to grasp or have levers instead of knobs are helpful as well.

Some apartment complexes have special "accessible" apartments. If the building doesn't have an elevator, a ground-floor apartment is needed.

RA can severely affect hand function as well. Many adaptive devices can help people with severe hand arthritis manipulate small objects. Specially designed eating utensils are available, but are relatively expensive. Many objects with small handles can be easily adapted with inexpensive equipment such as tubular foam. For example, the tubular foam can be cut to the desired length and then slipped over the handles of eating utensils, hand tools, pens, or pencils. With some creativity, even larger objects such as tennis rackets or golf clubs can be adapted for people with RA.

Numerous books, pamphlets, and websites are available that describe adaptive devices and home modifications that can help people with RA conserve energy and accomplish their activities of daily living with the least number of restrictions. Also, talk to your doctor about any problems that you are experiencing. He or she may recommend a home visit from a physical therapist or occupational therapist. These professionals can be very helpful in making recommendations to modify your home environment or suggesting adaptive devices.

65. What is the pneumococcal vaccine, and why do I need it?

The pneumococcal vaccine is a preparation of biological material that is injected into your body and causes your body to form antibodies to pneumococcus (plural = "pneumococci") bacteria. Whenever you are exposed to a particular type of bacteria, whether through an infection or via vaccination, your body produces antibodies to that bacterium. These antibodies then circulate in your bloodstream and can prevent—or at least lessen—the effects of future infections with that bacterium.

People with RA have approximately twice the risk of developing infections as compared with the risk for people without RA. Use of the pneumococcal vaccine has been shown to lower the risk of infections and complications from infections caused by pneumococci.

As mentioned previously in this book, people with RA have approximately twice the risk of developing infections as compared with the risk for the normal population (that is, people without RA). In particular, these patients are at risk for bacterial infections of the lung, such as bronchitis and pneumonia. One of the most common types of pneumonia is caused by the pneumococcal bacterium. Use of the pneumococcal vaccine has been shown to lower the risk of infections and complications from infections caused by pneumococci. Unfortunately, this vaccine is not effective in preventing the complications of pneumonias caused by other types of bacteria.

Studies of patients with RA who received the pneumococcal vaccine have demonstrated that this vaccination is both safe and effective. Vaccination does not result in disease flares or lead to deterioration of clinical and laboratory measures of RA disease activity.

According to the Advisory Committee on Immunization Practices, the pneumococcal vaccine is recommended for people who are older than 65 years of age and for people who are aged 2 to 64 and are at increased risk of getting pneumococcal pneumonia because of a long-term illness. All patients with RA should receive the pneumococcal vaccine, and should be encouraged to repeat the vaccination every five to six years.

66. Why do I need a flu vaccination?

Influenza infections can take a more severe course in people with RA. These infections are minor annoyances in the young and healthy, but can result in hospitalization and even death in elderly persons or individuals with a compromised immune system, like that found in RA. Many studies have demonstrated that influenza vaccinations can result in a significant decrease in infections and fewer complications of those infections when they do occur. Therefore influenza vaccinations are strongly recommended for patients with RA.

Studies of influenza vaccinations that included patients with RA showed that these individuals were able to take the vaccination safely. The vaccination of these patients resulted in the development of antibodies to the influenza virus similar to the antibodies found in persons without RA who received the same vaccine. Finally, the vaccinations in patients with RA did not result in a worsening of symptoms or a disease flare.

The flu vaccine is not associated with significant side effects. In people who are frail or elderly, there is an increased incidence of low fever and mild muscle aches that may last as long as 24 hours after a vaccination. Because the flu vaccine is made from only parts of the influenza virus, and because live viruses are not used in its preparation, you cannot develop influenza from the vaccine.

While the majority of patients with RA do get an influenza vaccination, approximately 30% do not. Reasons that people cite for not getting the vaccine include the following: they were never offered the vaccine, they were concerned about side effects, they did not believe the vaccine was effective, or they were not aware that they needed it. For the record: The flu vaccine is effective in preventing influenza; the vaccine is safe and will not result in disease flares; it is important for patients with RA to get the vaccine; and you will not get the "flu" from taking the influenza vaccine.

In contrast to the pneumococcal vaccine, which is given every five years, a new influenza vaccination must be administered every year. Each year, a new influenza virus becomes dominant and causes infections. The makers of the influenza vaccine try to predict which strains of influenza will be seen in a given year, select the most common influenza viruses, and make

The flu vaccine is effective in preventing influenza; the vaccine is safe and will not result in disease flares; it is important for patients with RA to get the vaccine; and you will not get the "flu" from taking the influenza vaccine.

them into a new vaccine. Thus a different vaccine is produced every year.

When you are inoculated with the current year's vaccine, you are immunized against those viruses that the vaccine makers believe will cause the most problems that year. The next year brings a new dominant influenza virus—and you need to get immunized against that one as well. Influenza vaccines are recommended every year for people with RA.

PART EIGHT

Osteoarthritis: The Basics

What is osteoarthritis?

What causes osteoarthritis?

How does osteoarthritis affect the joints?

More . . .

67. *What is osteoarthritis?*

Osteoarthritis (OA)

A type of arthritis characterized by pain and stiffness in the joints, such as those in the hands, hips, knees, spine, or feet; it is caused by the breakdown of cartilage.

Osteoarthritis is not an inevitable part of aging. Rather, it is believed to develop in any particular individual as a result of a combination of genetic susceptibility and environmental factors.

Osteoarthritis (OA) is a chronic condition that affects the joints. It occurs more frequently as we age. Of the more than 100 different types of arthritic conditions distinguished, OA is the most common, affecting more than 20 million people in the United States along. It is estimated that if everyone in the U.S. population who is older than age 65 underwent x-rays of their joints, more than half would show evidence of OA in at least one joint. While more than half of the population older than 65 may have OA, however, a large fraction will not. At one time OA was thought to be part of the normal aging process, but we now understand that this disease is not an inevitable part of aging. Rather, OA is believed to develop in any particular individual as a result of a combination of genetic susceptibility and environmental factors.

OA is characterized by inflammation and eventual loss of the cartilage in one or more joints. Cartilage is a complex substance composed of proteins and sugars that serves as a "shock absorber" between the bones of the joints. OA commonly affects the joints of the hands, feet, and spine, as well as the large weight-bearing joints, such as those in the hips and knees.

Symptoms of OA include joint pain, tenderness, decreased range of motion in the affected joints, and a variable amount of swelling and inflammation. OA is a progressive disease, meaning that the symptoms of pain and stiffness tend to worsen over time. The amount of pain and disability that any particular patient will experience is difficult to predict, however. Some patients have OA without symptoms, where the disease is found only incidentally on x-rays. Others have disease that can progress to serious disability and the need for surgery.

The term *osteoarthritis* is derived from a Latin term meaning "joint inflammation." Although the joints affected by OA may exhibit a small amount of inflammation, OA is not considered an inflammatory disease like rheumatoid arthritis (RA). Thus the term OA is technically inaccurate. Some alternative names have therefore been suggested for this condition, including osteoarthrosis, hypertrophic osteoarthritis, and **degenerative joint disease (DJD)**.

Although it is often referred to as a disease, OA is more appropriately called an arthritic condition that affects one or more joints. This condition results from a variety of disorders that lead to similar symptoms and joint changes. Rheumatologists separate patients with OA into two categories—primary and secondary—based on the cause of the arthritis:

- Most patients have **primary OA**. Primary OA suggests that the patient has no identifiable predisposing cause for the arthritis.
- Patients with **secondary OA** have an underlying cause for their joint symptoms, such as congenital hip dislocation, major trauma to the joint, joint infection, or a metabolic disease such as hemochromatosis or gout.

Clinically, it is generally not important to make a distinction between the two forms, because their treatment is similar.

68. What causes osteoarthritis?

Despite extensive research, scientists still do not know what causes OA. It is theorized that some type of cartilage damage starts a destructive process that, in genetically susceptible people, results in OA.

While the cause of OA is unknown, many factors are often associated with its development.

Aging

A person's risk for OA increases as he or she gets older, although OA can occur in younger patients, especially those with joint injuries or a history of joint disease (such as hip dysplasia).

Degenerative joint disease (DJD)

Joint destruction that occurs over a long period of time. This term is used synonymously with the term "osteoarthritis."

Primary osteoarthritis

The gradual breakdown of cartilage that occurs with age and is caused by stress on a joint.

Secondary osteoarthritis

Osteoarthritis that results from trauma to the joint or from chronic joint injury due to another type of arthritis, such as rheumatoid arthritis.

Ostheoarthritis: The Basics

Conversely, not every person in their seventies and eighties has OA. OA is not a normal part of the aging process.

Joint Injuries/Wear and Tear

OA occurs early in people who have experienced serious joint trauma, such as football players and ballet dancers. This condition is also encountered more frequently in people who perform heavy labor for a living, as compared to people who work in an office.

Inactivity

The joint cartilage requires frequent compression and re-laxation to remain healthy. This activity is believed to help circulate nutrients in the cartilage, which has no vascular sup-ply of its own. People who perform little or no exercise may note that their joints become stiff and painful. This tendency is thought to predispose them to OA.

Obesity

Excess weight puts undue stress on the weight-bearing joints of the body, adding to the wear and tear experienced by the joints. Surprisingly, obese people have an increased incidence of OA in non-weight-bearing joints, such as the fingers and shoulders. Scientists suggest that their fat tissue may release some chemical that predisposes these patients to OA, though this idea is just a theory at this point. Doctors recommend that people with OA try to reach their ideal weight by careful diet and exercise.

Genetics

There appears to be a genetic component to OA. For example, OA of the fingers occurs commonly in families and is most common in women.

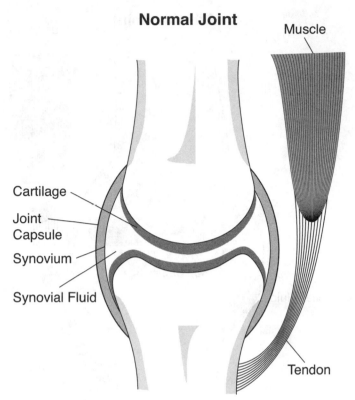

Figure 1 Normal joint.

While the cause of OA remains obscure, people who are at risk for OA, whether because of genetics or occupation, should take care to minimize their chance of developing this condition. To do so, they can participate in regular exercise (preferably low-impact exercise) and pay careful attention to their diet as a means of sustaining an ideal body weight.

69. How does osteoarthritis affect the joints?

OA is a disease of the joints. It predominantly affects the cartilage that lines the bones of the joint (**Figure 1**). Cartilage is the dense rubbery tissue that covers the ends of bones in a joint. In healthy people, its surface is smooth and slippery, which allows the bones in a joint to glide over one another easily. Cartilage also absorbs energy, like a shock absorber,

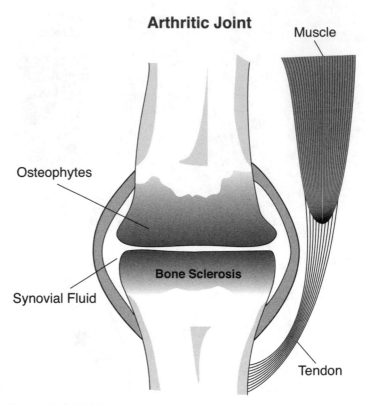

Figure 2 Arthritic joint.

from the jolts associated with movements such as walking. In OA, the cartilage of joints affected becomes inflamed and roughened and wears down. As the disease worsens, the cartilage can disappear completely, so that eventually one bone may rub against the next.

OA affects more than just the cartilage between the bones, however: It also affects the muscles, bones, ligaments and lining of the joint. The bones of the affected joint can undergo many changes. For example, small growths of bone, called **osteophytes** ("bone spurs"), can develop around the joints (**Figure 2**). These bone growths can lead to a knobby appearance and limit the motion of the joint. Small pieces of bone or cartilage may also break off and float inside the joint space, causing pain and

Osteophyte

An outgrowth of bone.

144

further damaging the surface of the cartilage. If a patient has OA of the spine, the bone spurs can press on nerves and cause numbness, tingling, or weakness in the arms or legs.

The bone that underlies the joint is called subchondral bone. In joints affected by OA, subchondral bone can become hardened and brittle and form cysts. In addition, the bone can lose its normal shape, in a process called **bone remodeling.** Scientists believe that subchondral bone remodeling plays an important role in the worsening of symptoms and is a common reason for joint replacements. Some new therapies for OA are aimed at inhibiting bone remodeling. For example, investigators are studying how drugs that are currently employed for the treatment of thinning bones (osteoporosis) will affect patients with OA. These drugs could potentially be used as disease-modifying agents in the treatment of OA.

When a joint affected by OA becomes painful, a person may become reluctant to exercise. As a result, the muscles surrounding the joint can become weak and thin from underuse. Without muscular support, the joint becomes less stable. This instability can lead to misalignment and increased wear on the joint, with resultant pain and disability. This cycle of pain, weakness, and worsening disease can be broken by use of pain medication and adherence to a regular exercise plan. If a painful joint keeps you from the activities you enjoy or from the exercise you need, speak to your doctor. He or she can offer a treatment that may help.

My finger, knee, and thumb joints get very stiff and even more uncomfortable in cool damp weather. Simple things like steering a car, opening bottles, and holding things become bothersome. I find that by using treatments like Tylenol, not carrying things that are heavy (over 5 pounds), and putting my luggage on wheels when traveling helps quite a bit. Also hand massages and warm towels on my hands and fingers help alleviate the discomfort.

—George

Bone remodeling

A cyclical process by which bone maintains a dynamic steady state through resorption and formation of a small amount of bone at the same site. Bone remodeling can occur as a result of joint disease.

When a joint affected by OA becomes painful, a person may become reluctant to exercise. The resulting cycle of pain, weakness, and worsening disease can be broken, however, by use of pain medication and adherence to a regular exercise plan.

Osteoarthritis: The Basics

70. What is cartilage?

Cartilage is a type of dense connective tissue. It is a tough, semitransparent, flexible tissue that is composed of cartilage cells (**chondrocytes**) and tough fibers that are surrounded by a dense material made of fats and protein (sort of like a fruit salad suspended inside a bowl of Jell-O). Among the many tissues affected by OA, cartilage is the most seriously damaged.

Chondrocyte

A cartilage cell.

In the joints, cartilage covers the surface of the bones and is referred to as **articular cartilage**. A dense fibrous membrane called the perichondrium covers this cartilage. The perichondrium helps to protect the cartilage from wear by allowing one bone to slide over another easily, which reduces friction and prevents damage. Additionally, the thick layer of cartilage found in weight-bearing joints, such as the hips and knees, acts as a shock absorber. In fact, cartilage can resist compressive forces up to 65 times body weight, which also helps to prevent injuries to the bones. Articular cartilage lacks an arterial blood supply and venous and lymphatic drainage. These additional tissues would compromise the cartilage's elasticity and toughness. Given that it does not have its own blood supply, the cartilage derives its nutrition primarily from the surrounding **synovial fluid** and, to a lesser extent, from the blood supply of the adjacent bone. As a consequence of this lack of vasculature, cartilage, once damaged, does not heal readily.

Articular cartilage

Tough, rubbery tissue that forms the surface of bones within joints.

Synovial fluid

A lubricating fluid secreted by the synovial membrane.

Cartilage's toughness and flexibility make it an ideal tissue for lining joints and providing mechanical support to many tissues in the body. For example, it forms part of the structure of the skeleton in the ribs, where it joins them to the breastbone (sternum). Cartilage is found in the tip of the nose, in the external ear, and in the walls of the windpipe (trachea) and the voice box (larynx), where it provides both support and shape. In a human embryo, the entire skeleton is made of cartilage. Even after we are born, many of our bones are little more than cartilage. As we grow and develop, however, these structures absorb calcium and phosphate, causing the bones to become hard and inflexible.

71. How does osteoarthritis affect the spine?

OA can affect a variety of joints in the body, including the spine. Like OA of the hips and knees, OA of the spine (sometimes called spondylitis) is a degenerative disease (**Figure 3**).

The spine is made up of many individual bones called vertebrae. Collectively, they provide a strong and flexible support for the body. The bones of the spine touch each other in an area in the back of the vertebrae called the facet joint. Like many other joints in the body, the facet joint is covered with cartilage. This cartilage allows the facet of the adjoining vertebra to easily slide over it. The vertebrae are separated from one another by intervertebral discs, which support the spine and provide additional flexibility and shock absorption when you are walking, running, or jumping. The vertebrae are connected to each other and to the muscles of the neck and back by a complex system of ligaments.

OA of the spine is one of the common causes of neck and back pain in people more than 50 years old. This disease affects the spine at the facet joints. Specifically, the cartilage covering these facet joints becomes inflamed and wears away. The inflammation leads to the development of small irregular growths of bone (called bone spurs or osteophytes) on the facet joints; eventually, bone spurs may form on the bodies of the vertebrae themselves.

These changes in the facet joints create additional mechanical pain on top of the pain resulting from the inflammation. Although the bone spurs do not directly cause pain, if they grow large enough, they can reduce the flexibility of the spine by interfering with the function of the facet joints. If they become large enough, they may press on the roots of the nerves

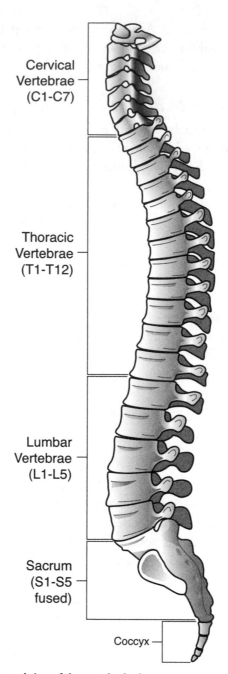

Cervical
Vertebrae
(C1-C7)

Thoracic
Vertebrae
(T1-T12)

Lumbar
Vertebrae
(L1-L5)

Sacrum
(S1-S5
fused)

Coccyx

Figure 3 Lateral view of the vertebral column.

as they leave the spine or may grow into the spinal canal and press on the spinal cord itself (a condition called spinal stenosis). Irritation of the nerve roots can result in numbness, tingling, or weakness of the hands or feet. Spinal stenosis can occur anywhere in the spine, but most commonly occurs in the neck or low back (lumbar spine). This condition can result in progressive pain and weakness that may affect the arms, legs, or even the bowel and bladder. In such a case, surgery is indicated to remove the bone growths; this treatment may bring about pain relief and return of function if the surgery is performed early enough in the course of the disease.

In the early stages of spinal OA, a person may not have any symptoms, though the disease may be evident on x-rays of the spine. Eventually, the affected individual may complain of mild neck or back pain and stiffness. The stiffness is usually worse in the morning or after sitting for long periods of time. Symptoms typically improve after a few minutes of moving around, but may worsen again at the end of the day. Symptoms can be slowly progressive and insidious. People with these symptoms slowly reduce their activity, resulting in weakened back muscles and more pain.

Engaging in low-impact exercise and stretching can improve symptoms. For example, exercising in a heated pool can help to relax tired muscles and decrease the impact on joints associated with running or walking.

OA has affected my spine more than any other part of my body. The disease caused the cartilage between the discs in my neck to wear away. This resulted in losing the function in my left arm. However, after two spinal fusions I now live a normal life with full use of my arm. I now play golf and swim. It is important to note that I am restricted in lifting heavy objects.

—George

Ostheoarthritis: The Basics

72. What are the risk factors for osteoarthritis?

The cause of OA is elusive in most cases. Nevertheless, physicians have noticed that certain groups have a higher rate of OA than others. You may find that you belong to one or more of these groups.

Age Greater Than 45 Years

Although OA risk increases with increasing age, not all people older than age 45 have degenerating cartilage in their knees and hips. The cartilage in patients with osteoarthritis looks different and has a different chemical composition when compared to "healthy" aged cartilage. Many experts now believe that OA is a disorder caused by a genetic susceptibility combined with injury to the joint. As we grow older, we accumulate more injuries to our joints, our ability to repair injured cartilage decreases, our weight tends to increase, and our chance of developing other forms of arthritis increases.

Female Sex

Women may have some unrecognized factor that predisposes them to accelerated cartilage wear, or perhaps women start out with thinner cartilage plates or have weaker supporting muscles or more lax supporting ligaments. Whatever the cause, women have a higher risk of developing OA. Before age 45, OA occurs more frequently in men; after age 55, it predominantly affects women. In the general population, the ratio of OA in men and women is 3:4.

Hereditary Conditions

Having certain hereditary conditions can predispose you to OA. These conditions include congenital hip dislocation, defective cartilage, and malformed joints. Conditions such as being knock-kneed or being bowlegged also increase the chances for wear and tear in the joint. Additionally, people who have close relatives with OA are at a higher risk for developing it themselves. This increased risk may be the result of a defect in the gene responsible for the formation of **collagen**, which is an important component of cartilage.

Ethnicity

The rate of OA is not the same for all ethnic groups. Indeed, both the rate of OA and the distribution of joints affected vary considerably across ethnic groups. In the United States, Caucasian Americans and African Americans have higher rates of OA than Hispanic Americans or members of other ethnic groups. The rate of knee OA in African Americans and Caucasian Americans is about the same, but the rate of OA of the hips is 33% higher in African Americans than in Caucasian Americans. In contrast, Asian Americans have a lower risk of hip OA than Caucasian Americans. Ethnic differences in the rates of OA may be explained by genetic factors that determine the height, weight, joint angles, amount of force, and other structural factors in the joints. Other genes that regulate the chemistry of joint cartilage may also account for these ethnic differences.

History of Joint Injuries

Joint injuries caused by physical activity or sports increases your risk of OA. Football players and ballet dancers, for example, are at higher risk for OA because of the stress that these activities place on their knees and hips. Swimmers and baseball players can suffer from OA of the shoulder or elbow for similar reasons.

Obesity

Obesity, which is defined as being 20% over one's healthy weight, is a known risk factor for OA. Being obese dramatically increases the stress on weight-bearing joints and accelerates degeneration once OA has started. Obese people commonly develop OA of the hips and knees, but they also have a higher risk of developing OA of the fingers. Some scientists have suggested that excess fat tissue causes increased cartilage inflammation even in non-weight-bearing joints.

Collagen

The major protein of connective tissue, cartilage, and bone.

Ostheoarthritis: The Basics

151

Other Arthritis

People who have another disease that affects the joints are at a higher risk for developing OA. Diseases such as rheumatoid arthritis, hemochromatosis, gout, and pseudogout, for example, can change the normal structure and function of cartilage and lead to early degeneration.

Education

As unlikely as it sounds, your level of education is associated with your risk of OA. Medical studies have found that the incidence of OA is highest in people with lower educational levels. One study, completed in 2000, demonstrated that college graduates had half the rate of OA as compared to those people who didn't graduate from high school. It is unlikely that reading and studying somehow make your joints healthier. Instead, college graduates may merely represent a different population of people from those without a high school diploma. College graduates, as a group, may have different ethnic backgrounds, have a lower ratio of women to men, and be less likely to be engaged in occupations that require physical labor as compared to people who didn't graduate from high school.

73. What is the prognosis for osteoarthritis?

In a worst-case scenario, a joint affected by OA can become stiff and painful. These symptoms result from the loss of the smooth, gliding surface that undamaged cartilage provides. As the disease progresses, the cartilage in a joint becomes thin and ragged, and more stiffness and a "catching" sensation may occur. These problems may cause a person to restrict the motion of that joint, which can in turn cause the surrounding ligaments to contract and tighten. The muscles that move the joint may ultimately become weakened and thin, with the overall effect being a loss of mobility and a disruption of work and recreation. This is a dire prediction, but not an unavoidable one: It reflects a scenario where the person with OA receives no medical care.

In reality, the prognosis for OA is generally very good. Many people ask, "Isn't rheumatoid arthritis the crippling arthritis—the type of arthritis that leads to disability?'" This question suggests that the prognosis for rheumatoid arthritis (RA) is bad, and the prognosis for all other types of arthritis is much better. This is an oversimplification. It is possible to have a mild case of RA or a severe case of OA. Moreover, many factors affecting the final outcome of arthritis depend on the person seeking treatment. Specifically, is the individual compliant with that treatment prescribed, is he or she receiving timely medical care, and does the individual work to maintain a healthy lifestyle?

It is difficult to predict the outcome of OA based on a history and physical exam. One person may have a relatively mild course of OA affecting a few joints; another may develop severe disease in many joints that render him or her unable to work. Some new studies suggest that "active synovitis" or inflammation of the cartilage seen on magnetic resonance imaging (MRI) or bone scan suggests a more aggressive and debilitating course of disease, although the results of these studies are still being debated. Some risk factors suggestive of a more disabling course of OA are believed to include obesity, early age of disease onset, sedentary lifestyle, traumatic joint injuries, and joint x-rays that show very little joint space or "bone-on-bone" contact between the bones of the joint.

Predicting the severity of anyone's OA is difficult. Nevertheless, identifying risk factors for progression of disease gives doctors and patients an opportunity to improve those risks that can be modified.

74. Is osteoarthritis an inherited disease?

Specialists in arthritic disease are often asked if OA is an inherited disease. People with OA are concerned about the possibility of their siblings developing the same problem or about their chances of "passing" the disease to their children.

The prognosis for osteoarthritis is generally very good.

Ostheoarthritis: The Basics

Studies of large populations of patients have demonstrated that OA does, indeed, have a major genetic component. Researchers have found that a pattern of heritability exists among joint sites. That is, if a parent has OA of the hip, there is a higher likelihood of his or her child having OA of the hip. Similar patterns have been identified for knee and spine OA. Unfortunately, the results across many studies are not always consistent. These discrepancies may arise because different investigators perform these studies a little differently. For example, they may use different populations of patients (older, younger, different ethnicities, and so on), different definitions of disease, and different ways of interpreting physical exams and x-rays. This complicates the task of understanding the complex genetics underlying OA.

Advances in DNA mapping have led arthritis specialists to examine the genetic makeup of individuals with OA to see if it differs from the genetic makeup of people without OA. Researchers in Asia have already identified variations in a gene responsible for the development of cartilage that is associated with a higher risk of hip and knee OA in Japanese and Chinese patients. This gene, which is called GDF5, was found to be more common in patients with OA than in a similar-size group of people without OA. These findings do not imply that GDF5 is the only gene that affects OA, however. The variations of the incidence of disease in populations affected, in the distribution of joints affected, and the inheritance pattern of this disease suggest that more than one gene may be involved and that other environmental factors may influence the onset and progression of OA.

To get a better understanding of the genetics of OA, an international research network has launched the largest study ever in an attempt to discover the source of the genetic susceptibility for OA. Scientists in the United States and the United Kingdom are studying families of people with OA. After taking detailed histories of patients, their family history of OA, and their risk factors for OA, these researchers will perform a complete physical exam of each patient, including x-rays of the hand, hip, knee, and lower spine. Next, blood samples will be taken for DNA testing. The researchers will then analyze the DNA samples and x-rays and chart the family tree in an attempt to identify the genes involved. If this study succeeds in pinpointing the gene or group of genes that cause OA, doctors may be able to identify those patients who are at risk for OA early and help them modify their lifestyles to slow the onset and reduce the symptoms of the disease. In the future, perhaps an effective treatment or a cure can be found with more modern genetic techniques.

Today, however, you should inform your doctor of any family history of OA. This information should include how the affected family members are related to you, which joints were affected, and how they were treated. For example, did that family member use a cane, take any specific medications, or have a joint replacement? This information will give your physician a better idea of your own risk for developing OA, including which joints may be affected and which risk factors you might be able to modify so as to reduce the impact of this disease.

75. What are the symptoms of osteoarthritis?

OA is principally a disease of the joints. As a consequence, its symptoms include pain, swelling, and stiffness of the joints.

The pain associated with OA usually has an insidious onset, is generally described as aching or throbbing, and may result from changes that have occurred over the last 15 to 20 years. It is usually worsened by activity and improved by rest. As the disease progresses and the joint becomes more damaged, the pain may become constant. This pain does not come from an irritation of the cartilage (which contains no nerves), but rather from the adjacent tissues that are stretched or inflamed.

Joint stiffness is another cardinal finding in OA. Morning stiffness can be found in all types of arthritis. This stiffness usually lasts about 30 minutes with OA, compared to an hour or more for rheumatoid arthritis. Many people with OA notice that their joints become stiff after they remain in the same position for long periods of time, such as after sitting or driving. Doctors sometimes call this type of stiffness "gelling." A few minutes of movement typically dispels this type of stiffness. The symptoms of stiffness can be improved by taking nonsteroidal anti-inflammatory drugs (NSAIDs), such as ibuprofen or indocin, or by taking a hot shower or bath.

Swelling of the joints is another classic feature of OA. It is caused by changes in the bone and fluid in the joint. The progressive destruction of the cartilage "cushion" leads to the release of chemicals that affect the bones of the joint. The ends of the bones can enlarge and form bony growths (bone spurs). These growths increase the appearance of joint enlargement or "knobbiness." An increase in the amount of joint fluid present also contributes to joint swelling. The erosion of cartilage results in an inflammation of the lining of the joint (called the **synovial membrane**). The synovial membrane produces excess fluid that collects in the joint, and this fluid production can increase with increased exercise or joint injury. As this fluid buildup can cause increased pressure and pain, doctors sometimes remove it to relieve symptoms.

Synovial membrane

Connective tissue that lines the cavity of a joint and produces synovial fluid.

OA typically affects the joints of the hand—principally the middle knuckle joints, the distal knuckle joints (next to the fingernail), and the base of the thumb. The hips, knees, feet (especially the big toe), neck, and low back are other common sites for OA. Finger joints affected by OA exhibit a hard bony swelling called **Heberden's nodes**. Sometimes early in the course of the disease there may be redness around the affected joint, similar to that seen with rheumatoid arthritis. Your doctor can usually tell the two types of arthritis apart, even without taking x-rays. In more advanced cases of OA,

Heberden's nodes

Knobby overgrowths of the joint nearest the fingertips in patients with osteoarthritis.

patients may experience a decreased range of motion in the affected joints.

Arthritis of the hip or knee affects a person's ability to get up or down from a seated position as a result of pain and stiffness. The change from sitting to standing puts more weight on your hips and knees than walking or standing; thus, the lower the seat, the harder it becomes to stand up. Many people describe great difficulty getting up, but after they are up they can walk. Purchasing chairs with higher seats and arm rests can help overcome this difficulty.

When OA strikes the spine, it can lead to pain and stiffness in the neck or low back. People with spinal OA complain of pain when they turn their heads or touch their toes. In addition, advanced spinal OA can produce bone spurs along the vertebrae. These bone spurs can pinch nerves along the spine, resulting in numbness and tingling of the hands or feet.

Secondary (indirect) problems created by OA include anxiety or depression, feelings of helplessness or dependence on others, and decreased ability to perform activities of daily living or work.

PART NINE

Diagnosing Osteoarthritis

How does a doctor make the diagnosis
of osteoarthritis?

Are bumps on the fingers a sign of osteoarthritis?

Does my doctor need to do x-rays
to diagnose osteoarthritis?

More . . .

76. How does a doctor make the diagnosis of osteoarthritis?

The diagnosis of osteoarthritis is made on the basis of your history and the results of your physical examination. There is no particular test whose results can be used to make a definitive diagnosis of OA.

Your doctor makes the diagnosis of OA on the basis of your history and the results of your physical examination. People with OA usually complain of pain, stiffness, or joint swelling, or some combination of these symptoms. During your physical exam, your doctor will pay special attention to your joints. He or she will check for swelling, tenderness, redness, joint effusions (fluid inside the joint), and your ability to flex and extend the affected joints. Your physician will also evaluate the distribution of affected joints. The pattern of distribution of inflamed joints varies according to the type of arthritis and can be an important clue in making a diagnosis of OA. For example, OA typically affects the middle knuckle joints, the distal knuckle joints (next to the fingernails), and the base of the thumb. The hips, knees, feet (especially the big toe), neck, and low back are other common sites for OA. In comparison, rheumatoid arthritis (RA) typically affects the wrists and the first knuckle joints of the hands; these joints are seldom affected by OA. Your doctor should look for other physical findings associated with OA, such as muscle wasting and weakness.

There is no particular test whose results can be used to make a definitive diagnosis of OA, so special tests such as blood tests and x-rays are usually not needed when this condition is suspected. Occasionally, your doctor may order one or more of these tests if he or she needs to exclude other arthritic conditions. Blood tests and radiographs may also be helpful for monitoring for side effects of medications or to help determine the extent of joint damage when considering surgical treatment.

77. Are bumps on the fingers a sign of osteoarthritis?

People with OA can develop swelling and redness around the joints of their fingers. Bumps around the farthest joints in your fingers (the ones farthest from your wrist) are called Heberden's nodes. They are typically about the size of a pea and are sometimes painful when they first develop, but frequently become less painful later. These knobby bumps are named after a British doctor, William Heberden, who worked in London at the time of the American Revolution.

Bumps around the next set of finger joints (the joints in the middle of the fingers) are called **Bouchard's nodes**. These nodes were first described by a French physician, Charles Joseph Bouchard, who worked in Paris during the nineteenth century. Bouchard's nodes occur less commonly than Heberden's nodes. Both types of nodes are caused by the same inflammatory process that causes swelling and pain in the hips and knees, and both are classic signs of OA.

Bouchard's nodes

Knobby overgrowths of the middle joint of the fingers in people with osteoarthritis.

Bouchard's and Heberden's nodes usually develop during middle age and begin with swelling and redness. The swelling is at first painful and tender; later, the redness goes away, and the pain and tenderness become less pronounced. The swelling is caused by inflammation of the cartilage in the finger joint. Eventually, small amounts of bone grow around the joint, leading to bone spurs. The nodes become hard and immovable. Infrequently, the nodes can become large enough to cause numbness in the fingertips and make it difficult to flex the fingers or make a fist. They may even cause the fingers to deviate sideways.

Heberden's nodes are more commonly found in women than in men. These nodes rarely require treatment, but if they reduce the functioning of the hand, surgery can help.

78. Does my doctor need to do x-rays to diagnose osteoarthritis?

When a person presents to a physician with complaints of joint pain and swelling, the doctor understands that numerous conditions could cause these symptoms. The history you

Diagnosing Osteoarthritis

provide and the results of your physical exam may point to one or more diagnoses. It is helpful to have further evidence to help clarify one diagnosis and eliminate others. Therefore, it is appropriate to perform x-rays on any swollen and painful joint to help determine the cause of these symptoms.

People with OA have characteristic changes in the joints that can be seen on an x-ray. These changes include an uneven loss of cartilage in the joint, called "loss of joint space" on the x-ray interpretation. Small growths of bone (bone spurs) may develop around the joints, and the bone underneath the cartilage may become thickened or hardened (bony sclerosis). In addition, the bone may change shape and develop cysts. In the early stages of OA, these bone changes may appear on x-rays, but the patient may not experience any pain or swelling.

Although x-rays cannot conclusively confirm the presence of OA, they can be a useful tool for distinguishing between OA and rheumatoid arthritis, gout, and other conditions. Additionally, x-rays establish a baseline for comparison. As the disease progresses, they can be used to monitor changes in the bones over time. Often, as part of a person's initial evaluation with a rheumatologist, chest x-rays are ordered in addition to x-rays of any swollen joints. Chest x-rays are performed to evaluate the lungs for diseases that are sometimes associated with arthritis.

X-rays are usually performed in a special hospital department (Radiology) by a radiologic technician or a radiographer, who will tell you which part of your body is to be x-rayed. These technicians are highly skilled. They must have college degrees, undergo additional training, and pass a state licensing examination before they can take x-rays. These technician's training is different from that of the radiologist—a radiologist is a physician who is trained to interpret x-ray images.

To make the image, x-rays are passed through your body and captured on special film. This film is then developed and examined. Standard x-rays are particularly good at showing abnormalities of the bone, but they rarely show problems in soft tissues. For this reason, they do not show the changes associated with early-stage arthritis very well. Despite this drawback, x-rays can highlight areas that help the doctor to diagnose arthritis, such as damaged areas on the bone.

I am not certain about diagnosis not concerning the spine. In my case MRI's were performed to confirm the diagnoses and pinpoint the areas in the neck and spine that were causing the pain.

—George

Diagnosing Ostheoarthritis

PART TEN

Treatment of Osteoarthritis

Is it important to learn more about my osteoarthritis?

What are some medical treatments for osteoarthritis?

What are nondrug treatments for
osteoarthritis-related pain?

More . . .

79. Is it important to learn more about my osteoarthritis?

Learning more about your own disease will help you better understand why your doctor recommends certain treatments and asks you to avoid others. It will also help you feel in control of your osteoarthritis and lead you to become an active participant in your own care.

While you don't have to get a medical degree, learning more about your own disease will help you better understand why your doctor recommends certain treatments and asks you to avoid others. In addition, knowing more about your disease will help you feel in control of your OA and lead you to become an active participant in your own care.

There are many things that you can learn about OA, such as how it starts, what makes it worse, and what can help to reduce joint pain and impairment. In one study of adults who were provided with a self-help educational program, doctors found that even four years later, those patients who had completed the educational program had more knowledge of OA, had less joint pain, and tended to comply more with recommended therapies, compared with similar patients who didn't participate in the educational program.

The Arthritis Foundation sponsors an arthritis self-help course, which is intended to teach people with OA about the latest pain management techniques, the newest medications, and the best ways to manage stress and fatigue. You can learn more about this program by calling your local chapter of the Arthritis Foundation or going on the Internet and looking at the following website: http://www.arthritis.org/events/getinvolved/ProgramsServices/ArthritisSelfHelp.asp.

It is most definitely important to learn more. This is a progressive disease; we need to understand how this works, what to expect, how to deal and live with it. It is also extremely important to understand that new treatments and drugs are constantly being utilized. The more you learn the better you will be able to manage it and enjoy life.

—George

80. What are some medical treatments for osteoarthritis?

Osteoarthritis is the most common type of arthritis. Although it cannot be cured, its symptoms—such as pain, stiffness, and swelling—can usually be managed effectively. Doctors try to achieve this goal with the least amount of medication possible and with the safest medications possible.

Regular exercise is very helpful in relieving symptoms and preventing disease progression; maintaining a normal body weight is also important in this regard. Aerobic exercise and exercises to strengthen the quadriceps (a large muscle in the front of the thigh) are particularly helpful for treating OA of the knee or hip.

Likewise, walking aids such as canes are helpful in the management of hip and knee OA. These devices decrease pain by reducing the weight placed on an arthritic hip or knee. Their use allows for increased physical activity.

Regular exercise is very helpful in relieving symptoms and preventing disease progression; maintaining a normal body weight is also important.

If you use a cane, you should hold it in the hand opposite the knee or hip that is hurting. For example, if your right knee hurts, hold the cane in your left hand. Some people associate the use of a cane with age and disability. Those people may choose to use a cane selectively—for example, when they know they will be walking some distance, as in a fairground or shopping mall. Using the cane this way can alleviate flare ups of discomfort both during and after the activity.

Taping of the patella can be helpful for relieving some types of knee pain. A wide variety of different knee braces can also be very helpful in such cases. A physical therapist can assist you in deciding whether any of these treatments are right for you. Many of these treatments have been discussed elsewhere in this book as well.

Treatment of Ostheoarthritis

If medication is necessary, then the safest drugs should be selected first. Many people will do well taking acetaminophen (brand name: Tylenol). Although this drug is not an anti-inflammatory medication, for many people it is an effective treatment for pain. Unlike many prescription medications, acetaminophen is inexpensive, readily available, and relatively safe. The side effects most commonly associated with acetaminophen include nausea, constipation, and occasionally drowsiness. The most worrisome side effect is liver toxicity, though this problem is exceedingly rare when acetaminophen is taken as directed.

If acetaminophen doesn't work or doesn't work well enough, a nonsteroidal anti-inflammatory drug (NSAID) can be tried. These medications are available both in over-the-counter formulations and in higher doses by prescription from your doctor. The side effects most commonly encountered with this class of medication are upset stomach and ulcer complications. The risk of stomach ulcers is greatest in those individuals who have acid reflux disease, use corticosteroids, smoke tobacco, or drink alcohol. Those persons who are at highest risk for ulcer disease may need to take additional medications such as cimetidine (Tagamet) or omeprazole (Prilosec) to help protect their stomachs against these side effects. Misoprostol (Cytotec) can also be used to protect the stomach, but it produces upset stomach symptoms as well, so it is not used frequently for this purpose. Unfortunately, the need to protect the stomach increases the number of pills that must be taken—and hence the cost of treatment.

Taking NSAIDs is also associated with a risk of damage to your kidneys. This risk is greatest in people who are older than 65, individuals with hypertension or congestive heart failure, or those taking diuretics or angiotensin-converting enzyme (ACE) inhibitors. Patients who are on anticoagulation therapy, such as those taking warfarin (Coumadin) or heparin, should also use NSAIDs with caution.

Members of a newer type of NSAID class, called COX-2 inhibitors (such as Celebrex), have received a lot of attention recently. These medications have a little less risk of serious stomach complications such as ulcers, but they are much more expensive than the older NSAIDs, and their safety advantage for the stomach is cancelled out if you take even a small dose of aspirin. Two other COX-2 inhibitors, named Vioxx and Bextra, were removed from the market because they were associated with an increased risk of heart disease. For these reasons, this type of medication offers only a small advantage for a limited number of people with OA.

Older NSAIDs called nonacetylated salicylates (e.g., salsalate, trilisate) are a good choice for some people, especially those who have experienced stomach upset with other NSAIDs or those who have decreased kidney function. These medications are relatives of aspirin, although they are chemically different than regular aspirin. Nonacetylated salicylates are inexpensive and are less likely to cause upset stomach or kidney problems than many other NSAIDs. They can cause ringing in the ears, difficulty hearing, or dizziness if their levels in the blood become too high, but these side effects disappear quickly if the medication is temporarily stopped.

Many people with OA are intolerant of the side effects of NSAIDs or still have pain despite treatment with these drugs. For these people, physicians may prescribe narcotic pain medications, such as codeine, morphine, or synthetic morphine derivatives (e.g., hydrocodone, oxycodone). These medications have no anti-inflammatory effects but can treat pain very effectively. They are unlikely to cause ulcers, but can cause upset stomach, drowsiness, constipation, or other side effects. Some people believe that there is a stigma attached to taking pain medications, and many worry—unnecessarily—about becoming "addicted" to pain medication. If you are taking a narcotic painkiller on a regular basis, it is appropriate to be under the care of a pain specialist. A pain specialist can help

If you are taking a narcotic painkiller on a regular basis, it is appropriate to be under the care of a pain specialist. A pain specialist can help to maximize your pain relief while avoiding the side effects and dependency linked to these medications.

Treatment of Ostheoarthritis

to maximize your pain relief while avoiding the side effects and dependency linked to these medications.

Marijuana has a long history of medicinal use. For millennia, many cultures have used preparations of this herb to treat pain. In the United States, marijuana was widely used for this purpose as late as the 1800s. Several studies have found that marijuana does, indeed, have analgesic effects. In fact, the active ingredient in marijuana, called tetrahydrocannabinol (THC), may work as well in treating cancer pain as the narcotic medication codeine. When given to patients taking opiate pain medications, marijuana seems to enhance the pain relief associated with those medications, which could allow for the use of lower doses of opiate pain relievers in patients suffering from chronic pain. Scientists and pain specialists are currently developing new medications based on marijuana to treat pain.

To be clear, marijuana is an illegal substance in the United States. In June 2005, the U.S. Supreme Court ruled, in a 6-3 decision, that people whose doctors have prescribed marijuana for medical purposes can be arrested and prosecuted, overriding medicinal marijuana statutes in ten states. In their decision, the members of the Court emphasized that their ruling was not based on whether marijuana is effective for pain relief.

Viscosupplementation

A treatment option for people with osteoarthritis of the knee that involves the injection of hyaluronan, a natural component of synovial fluid, directly into the knee joint.

Corticosteroid injections can be very helpful in OA, and sometimes **viscosupplementation** injections (e.g., Hyalgan, Synvisc) can relieve knee pain if nothing else works. When pain is constant and medications and other conservative treatments offer little relief, surgical treatment should be considered. Pain and limited mobility should not be accepted as "part of the disease process." Discuss your pain with your doctor, and seek out the best therapy together.

I have had some good results from acupuncture in the early stages. Also I found massages of the hands and feet help, as well as hot wax treatment for my hands and fingers.

—George

81. What are nondrug treatments for osteoarthritis-related pain?

Pain can be the predominant symptom in OA, and it is a major cause of the disability associated with this type of arthritis. Your doctor should assess the level of pain that you have at each meeting and determine how much this pain is affecting your ability to function. This assessment provides a rational basis for a pain treatment program. Your doctor should teach you about pain, pain management options, and self-management programs as part of any OA treatment plan.

OA pain is traditionally treated with nonsteroidal anti-inflammatory drugs (e.g., ibuprofen, naproxen) if it is of moderate intensity, or with medications from the opiate family (e.g., demerol, morphine, hydrocodone) if it is severe. But what if these medications are not controlling the pain and surgery is not an option? What other options are available?

Experts in pain management recognize that pain is not simply the result of a physical problem, but has psychological and social dimensions, too. Addressing all of these areas is important when treating pain.

A group of therapies, collectively known as cognitive-behavioral therapy (CBT), addresses the physiologic, psychological, and social dimensions of pain. In fact, current research supports the use of CBT as an effective means to reduce pain and improve function in OA. CBT is based on the idea that thought and behavior patterns can worsen the perception of pain and contribute to feelings of helplessness and fatigue. These feelings can be significant obstacles to recovery. The goal of CBT, then, is to alter the way you think and behave when you feel pain. CBT is not a single treatment, but rather a group of treatments, each of which employs a different modality to reduce pain—for example, stress management, relaxation techniques, and cognitive restructuring.

Both anxiety and stress have negative effects on patients with OA. Pain and its accompanying disability can increase a person's stress level. Conversely, stresses from work, family, or the environment can increase a person's perception of pain. Stress management is used to break this cycle of stress and pain and minimize a patient's response to stress. First, you learn to recognize those situations or occurrences that trigger stress. Once identified, you can learn to avoid these stressful conditions. When avoidance isn't possible, relaxation training may provide relief. Relaxation training can take the form of biofeedback, progressive relaxation exercises, or guided imagery. All of these techniques can reduce muscle tension, which can in turn aggravate pain, and allow you a chance to shift your attention away from your pain, which reduces your perception of pain.

Cognitive-behavioral therapy is an important and effective therapy that can reduce pain and psychological disability and enhance a person's self-efficacy and pain coping skills. It should be integrated with other treatments in a multi-disciplinary approach to the treatment of osteoarthritis.

Negative thoughts that are associated with pain are often erroneous and distorted, but can nevertheless worsen your pain and increase your emotional distress. Cognitive restructuring is a technique that attempts to deal with this problem. Patients are taught to identify the negative thoughts that enter the mind when they experience pain. For example, you might think, "This pain is the worst I've ever felt. I'll never get better. Maybe there's something else the matter with me, like cancer." A therapist can help you first challenge the validity of these thoughts and then modify them. For example, you might tell yourself, "I've had this kind of pain before and got better in a few hours" or "This pain is bad, but I haven't had a flare in a month since starting my exercise program. I'm really getting better."

CBT is an important and effective therapy that can reduce pain and psychological disability and enhance a person's self-efficacy and pain coping skills. This does not imply that you should replace all of the more common pain treatments with CBT, but rather that this technique should be integrated with other treatments in a multidisciplinary approach to the treatment of OA.

82. Can a change in diet improve or reverse osteoarthritis?

Many claims are made that changes in diet can prevent, improve, or reverse the symptoms of OA. These diets suggest eliminating your consumption of red meats, "acidic" foods (such as tomatoes and peppers), fatty foods (red meat and dairy products), processed sugar, or alcohol. Proponents of these diets contend that these substances cause "allergies" or other immune reactions, which are manifested as OA. Other diets recommend adding certain foods to treat OA, such as fish oils, green vegetables, seaweed, seeds, and whole grains. These foods are thought to contain micronutrients, antioxidants, and other substances that will prevent the onset of OA. Still other diets promote regular fasting as a way of "cleansing the body" and decreasing the amount of immunological irritants one takes in.

Currently, medical research does not support the concept that modifying your diet or eating larger amounts of certain foods will prevent OA or reverse its effects. Additionally, the regular consumption of "acidic" foods is not associated with an increased risk of OA. While the use of moderate amounts of alcohol and tobacco are not recommended as a general rule, their consumption has not been associated with increased rates of OA.

Despite these facts, diet is an important part of a healthy lifestyle, and research suggests that some changes in diet may be helpful when you have OA. Specifically, the goals of a healthy diet in individuals with OA should be to treat obesity and osteoporosis.

Overweight persons might reduce their chances for developing or aggravating their osteoarthritis by losing weight. Obesity increases the risks associated with most types of surgery and makes rehabilitation following orthopedic surgery more difficult. Furthermore, if a person already has osteoarthritis

Diet is an important part of a healthy lifestyle. The goals of a healthy diet in individuals with osteoarthritis should be to treat obesity and osteoporosis.

Treatment of Ostheoarthritis

in a weight-bearing joint, having a higher body weight can accelerate the joint damage. Therefore, a diet low in calories can ameliorate at least this risk factor.

The principal mineral in bones is calcium; vitamin D is necessary for the body to absorb and use calcium. People with low calcium and vitamin D intakes can suffer from osteoporosis, which is itself a risk factor for OA. Specialists in the treatment of osteoporosis recommend exercise and adequate calcium intake, as recommended for age and gender, to help maintain bone density. In addition, supplementation with vitamin D can help prevent bone loss. In particular, vitamin D deficiency has been shown to increase a person's risk for OA disease progression. Although supplementation of vitamin D in patients with normal vitamin D levels has not been shown to decrease the rate of OA progression, taking the recommended daily requirement of this vitamin is not associated with adverse events.

83. Can losing weight improve my osteoarthritis symptoms?

Obesity is a risk factor for OA. It causes increased force across weight-bearing joints, which can contribute to cartilage breakdown and, therefore, to OA. As compared to non-obese people, obese individuals are more likely to develop OA in both knees or in both hips rather than in just one knee or one hip. Interestingly, obesity increases this risk not only for weight-bearing joints such as the knees and hips, but also for non-weight-bearing joints such as the hands. Scientists aren't sure how obesity contributes to OA of the hands, but studies have shown that obese individuals are more likely to develop it.

Body mass index (BMI) is a popular way of evaluating obesity. Your BMI is calculated using a simple formula that takes into account your height in centimeters and your weight in kilograms. Values of about 18.5 to 25 are considered normal;

higher numbers indicate overweight or obesity. Having a body mass index in the range of 30–35 increases your risk of developing OA of the knee by four to five times.

If you are overweight, losing weight may help to slow the progression of OA, especially in weight-bearing joints. In addition, weight loss may postpone the need for hip or knee joint replacement. If such surgery is needed, it is likely to have fewer complications in people who are not overweight.

84. Can exercise improve my osteoarthritis symptoms?

Exercise is an excellent therapy for most people with OA. Exercise increases your endurance, muscle strength, and range of motion, and decreases your joint pain. Additionally, it lowers your weight and decreases your risk for high blood pressure, diabetes, and heart disease.

The benefits of exercise in OA are especially evident with low-impact, weight-bearing exercises such as walking, biking, swimming, or water aerobics. Exercise equipment such as a treadmill, elliptical glider, or stationary bike can be helpful in this regard as well.

Before beginning any exercise program, you should consult with your doctor. He or she will advise you on the risks associated with the exercise. Your doctor should not only discuss the risks and benefits to your joints, but also include information about other risks associated with exercise, such as those associated with falls or heart attacks.

It makes good sense to start every exercise session with some slow stretching exercises to warm up. A regimen of low-impact exercise that emphasizes increased range of motion is ideal. For example, tai chi or an active range of motion and relaxation program such as "range of motion dance" can help relieve stiffness and improve function. Water exercise is also

The benefits of exercise in osteoarthritis are especially evident with low-impact, weight-bearing exercises such as walking, biking, swimming, or water aerobics.

Treatment of Ostheoarthritis

helpful, especially for people with more advanced arthritis of the hip or knee who would not be able to tolerate conventional exercising in a gym. High-impact exercises such as basketball or volleyball are not a good idea if you have arthritis of the spine, hips, knees, ankles, or feet. The Arthritis Foundation offers exercise classes designed for people with arthritis called PACE (People with Arthritis Can Exercise); contact your local chapter to find out more about these classes.

Mild muscle aches or stiffness after starting an exercise program is normal. If you experience one of these problems, rest for a few days and then try resuming the exercise program at a lower intensity and for a shorter length of time. Over time, you should be able to gradually increase the length of time and the intensity of your exercise program. If exercising leads to severe joint pain, joint swelling, or redness, then you should modify your exercise program. If you are having difficulty finding the right exercise program for use at home or the gym, consult a physical therapist. He or she can help create the most appropriate exercise program for you.

85. Is night pain common in osteoarthritis?

The joint pain associated with OA typically gets worse during exercise and improves with rest. However, when OA is advanced and joints are significantly damaged, patients may experience pain while resting—especially pain at night that keeps them from sleeping. This problem can lead to daytime sleepiness, irritability, clouded thoughts, and depression.

Night pain associated with OA occurs predominantly in the hips and shoulders. It is aggravated by overuse of the joints and improves with several days rest. Individuals who suffer from night pain can benefit from some simple strategies, however.

People with night pain should identify those activities that cause or worsen their night pain, and then avoid or modify these activities so as to reduce the stress on joints. Such modifications might include using a cane when walking, using a motorized wheelchair if walking is too difficult, or using a "grabber" to pick up objects and reduce the amount of back bending necessary.

Use of a firm mattress that distributes the body weight evenly over a large area can also offload pressure on the affected joint. Newer, foam-based mattresses may offer advantages in this regard. Placing pillows between the knees or under the arm may also help to relieve OA-related pain, as may elevating the entire leg with a pillow. You should avoid placing a pillow under the knee so that the knee is flexed for long periods of time, however. Prolonged flexion of the inflamed knee can lead to a contracture of the ligaments and a reduced ability to fully extend the knee. If necessary, you can also try a variety of sleep positions.

If pain persists, taking pain medication before going to sleep may help you to get a good night's rest. Appropriate medications may include nonsteroidal anti-inflammatory drugs (e.g., ibuprofen), narcotic medications (e.g., morphine or hydrocodone), or even antidepressants (e.g., amitriptyline), all of which have been shown to be effective in relieving chronic pain conditions. You should discuss the type and dosage of nighttime medications with your doctor before taking them.

In some cases, night pain caused by OA may be very difficult to endure. Intractable pain may be a sign that it is time to consider surgery.

I experience night pain in my knee and fingers, but not on a regular basis. It seems to happen when I have tried to do too much during the day. Only rarely does it interfere with my sleep.

—George

Night pain caused by osteoarthritis may sometimes be very difficult to endure. Intractable pain may be a sign that it is time to consider surgery.

Treatment of Ostheoarthritis

86. Can osteoarthritis-related foot pain be improved with shoe inserts?

Your foot is a complex structure that includes 26 bones and 33 separate joints. Even in people without OA, foot pain is often difficult to avoid due to the large weight-bearing load placed on the feet. Foot pain in OA is not an unusual symptom. As in the hips, knees, and fingers, OA may affect the cartilage of any or all of the small joints in the feet, resulting in pain and limitation of function. After many years, small fragments of cartilage can come loose and float inside the joints of the foot, which in turn can worsen pain and inflammation. Eventually, the cartilage can erode completely away, so that the bones begin to rub together.

The symptoms of OA of the foot are insidious. They can begin slowly, such that the person experiences minor pain and swelling after extended periods of standing or walking. As the disease progresses and the cartilage wears out, the pain can become intense and seriously impair a person's mobility.

Rheumatologists and orthopedists often suggest that patients with OA of the foot wear sneakers. The insole of a sneaker is made of soft, shock-absorbent material. This kind of padding can cushion the impact associated with walking and help to preserve the knee and foot joints.

Orthotics are devices that fit into shoes and correct foot-related problems. Like sneakers, they can absorb shocks and redistribute pressure so that foot joints are less painful. In-shoe orthotics can be fashioned with a lateral wedge. This wedge, which is made of a firm but flexible material, can help to align the knee joint and take pressure off the medial (inside) portion of the knee joint.

If you have foot or knee pain, in-shoe orthotics may ease your pain and decrease the stress on your joints. Unfortunately, people with diabetes, poor circulation, or swelling can have problems when using orthotics. Your rheumatologist, orthopedist, or podiatrist can evaluate you and determine whether you might benefit from an orthotic.

I am just starting to experience foot pain. It seems to be very bad upon waking and for several minutes after then goes away. Inserts have been recommended but have not tried them yet.

—George

87. What are glucosamine and chondroitin sulfate?

Glucosamine and chondroitin sulfate are both substances that are found naturally in the body. A glucosamine molecule is formed by adding an amino group (NH_2) to a glucose molecule, thereby creating an amino sugar. Glucosamine is a component of a number of structures in the body and is believed to play a role in the formation and repair of cartilage.

Chondroitin sulfate is a member of a class of large molecules called sulfated glycosaminoglycans; these molecules contain sugars, proteins, and sulfur. Chondroitin sulfate is a major constituent in various connective tissues, as well as bone, and cartilage. It is thought to impart elasticity to cartilage.

Both glucosamine and chondroitin sulfate are sold as nutritional supplements. Manufacturers of these supplements extract their raw materials from animal tissue. For example, glucosamine can be extracted from the shells of shrimp, lobsters, or crabs, while chondroitin sulfate can be removed from the cartilage of animals, such as sharks.

88. Do glucosamine and chondroitin sulfate work for osteoarthritis?

Glucosamine and chondroitin sulfate supplements are very popular treatments for OA. Unfortunately, robust scientific evidence that demonstrates their effectiveness in treating this condition is lacking.

Glycosaminoglycans are the building blocks for cartilage. Glucosamine is a precursor to a glycosaminoglycan; chondroitin sulfate is the most common glycosaminoglycan found in human cartilage. The rationale for taking these supplements is the belief that they might help to build new cartilage, repair OA-related damage, or slow the progression of new damage. To date, these purported effects have consisted largely of hopeful speculation, though this speculation has prompted many scientific trials of these supplements.

Unfortunately, the studies performed so far have been of poor quality. Most included only a small number of patients and had a very short duration. Furthermore, many of these studies were underwritten by manufacturers of the supplements (a conflict of interest). Perhaps not surprisingly, the manufacturer-sponsored studies seemed to come up with rosier conclusions than larger, more recent, and more objective studies. As a result, the earlier studies are of limited value when we try to judge the effectiveness of a treatment for a disease that affects millions of people and lasts for many years.

In response to the popularity of these supplements and the lack of good science supporting their use, a branch of the National Institutes of Health undertook a study to see how these dietary supplements affected OA. This study, which was called the Glucosamine/Chondroitin Arthritis Intervention Trial (GAIT), was the first large-scale, multicenter clinical trial in the United States to test the effects of glucosamine hydrochloride (glucosamine) and sodium chondroitin sulfate (chondroitin sulfate) for treatment of knee OA. The study investigated whether glucosamine and chondroitin sulfate, when used either separately or in combination, reduced pain in patients with knee OA. It reached the following conclusion:

Glucosamine and chondroitin sulfate alone or in combination did not reduce pain *[emphasis added] effectively in the overall group of patients with osteoarthritis of the knee. Exploratory analyses suggest that the combination of glucosamine and chondroitin sulfate* may *[emphasis added] be effective in the subgroup of patients with moderate-to-severe knee pain.*

As discouraging as those results were, many people remain motivated to try these supplements. Patients believe that these supplements are relatively inexpensive and safe. Moreover, many are frustrated with a lack of improvement of their pain from their prescription medications and want to avoid knee replacement surgery.

If you think you might benefit from these supplements or have questions about their risks and benefits, it's worthwhile to discuss this topic with your doctor.

89. Can diacerhein help my osteoarthritis?

Diacerhein is one of the anthraquinones. Anthraquinones are organic compounds derived from plants and animals. They occur naturally in some plants, such as aloe and senna, as well as in fungi, lichens, and insects. Anthraquinones serve as a basic skeleton for these organisms' pigments. Humans have used these substances for centuries for their laxative properties as well as for the production of dyes.

Recently, diacerhein has been used for the treatment of OA by practitioners of alternative medicine. In animal studies, these compounds have been shown to have anti-inflammatory properties as well as a protective effect on cartilage. It is not yet clear whether diacerhein is both safe and effective in humans, however.

Investigators have reviewed seven studies that enrolled people with OA who were treated with diacerhein. These studies included 2069 patients with OA who received diacerhein; these individuals were compared to another group of patients with OA who were treated with a placebo (i.e., sugar pills). When investigators evaluated the group treated with diacerhein, they found that those patients had a statistically significant decrease in pain in the hips and knees. When x-rays of the patients' hips were compared, researchers found a statistically significant slowing of the progression of OA. Evaluations of knee x-rays did not show this benefit. The most frequent adverse event experienced by patients in the diacerhein-treated group was diarrhea.

Overall, for the treatment of OA, these studies demonstrated a small, consistent benefit from taking diacerhein. The long-term effects of taking this compound have not been examined.

90. Is hyaluronic acid an effective treatment for osteoarthritis?

Hyaluronic acid is a clear jelly-like material that is found in many places in the body, including the synovial fluid of joints and the vitreous humor of the eyes. Hyaluronic acid acts as a binding, lubricating, and protective agent and may boost the shock-absorbing properties of a person's joints.

Recognizing hyaluronic acid's many functions in the body, scientists have looked for ways to use it to treat disease. Hyaluronic acid was first used in eye surgery to replace lost vitreous fluids. Today, it is used in plastic surgery to improve the appearance of scars and wrinkles. In this application, Restylane (the brand name for hyaluronic acid) is injected into the skin to "puff up" tissues.

Rheumatologists and orthopedic surgeons have used hyaluronic acid injections to treat the knees of people affected by OA, a type of treatment sometimes called viscosupplementation. The addition of this material to the joints provides a cushioning and lubrication effect. In addition, hyaluronic acid injections provide pain relief even after the medication is no longer detectable in the joint. These injections are an alternative to corticosteroid ("cortisone") injections for people with knee pain that is not manageable with physical therapy and pills.

Hyaluronic acid is not absorbed through the skin, and it cannot be given orally because it is digested by stomach enzymes. Treatment for OA requires a weekly injection into the knee for three to five consecutive weeks, depending on the brand used and based on the doctor's judgment. This type of treatment has several advantages and disadvantages in comparison to cortisone injections. The main advantage is that the pain relief it produces might last longer than the pain relief offered by a cortisone injection. Unfortunately, hyaluronic acid injections may take a little bit longer to work than cortisone injections, and this therapy requires a greater number of visits and injections. Finally, hyaluronic acid injections are much more expensive than cortisone injections. For this reason, hyaluronic acid is recommended primarily as a last alternative before pursuing surgery.

Recently, some placebo-based, controlled studies have cast doubt on the efficacy of hyaluronic acid injections. You should discuss the results of these studies with your doctor and decide whether this therapy is right for you.

91. Can the osteoporosis drug risedronate help treat osteoarthritis?

Risedronate (brand name: Actonel) is a **bisphosphonate**—a type of drug that is used to treat thinning of the bones (osteoporosis). Other drugs in this category include alendronate (Fosamax) and ibandronate (Boniva). Risedronate is also under investigation as a treatment for OA.

Bisphosphonate
One of a class of drugs used to maintain or improve bone density.

The results of a recent British study of middle-aged men and women with OA of the knee suggest that risedronate may slow the progression of OA and improve pain symptoms. In

Treatment of Ostheoarthritis

this study, patients with OA of the knee, all of whom had pain, stiffness, and crepitus (the grinding sensation you get when bending an arthritic joint), were separated into three groups. The control group was given a placebo (sugar pill), the second group was given a low dose of risedronate (5 milligrams), and the third group was given a high dose of risedronate (15 milligrams). These treatments were continued over the course of a year and were accompanied by regular physical examinations for pain and stiffness as well as x-rays of the knee looking for signs of joint destruction and cartilage thickness.

The researchers found that those patients who were treated with the highest dose of risedronate (15 milligrams) experienced improvements in pain, stiffness, and disability and had less of a need for walking aids. An examination of the x-rays revealed that these patients also had less joint destruction than members of the other two treatment groups.

While these results came from only one small study, they do offer hope that the use of high-dose risedronate might slow joint destruction and delay the need for joint replacement surgery in patients with knee OA. Currently, risedronate is not FDA approved for the treatment of OA. You should discuss the risks and benefits of this treatment with your physician before trying it.

92. I've heard that an antibiotic can help osteoarthritis. Is that true?

It is true that an antibiotic—doxycycline—has been evaluated in the treatment of OA. In studies employing animal models of OA, this drug has been shown to prevent or slow the progression of OA. It is theorized that doxycycline can decrease the amount of cartilage-degrading enzymes found around the joints.

The results in human trials were equivocal, however, and doxycycline had not shown much promise for OA in the past.

However, a recently published medical study offers some hope. In this study, obese women with OA-related pain in one knee took 200 milligrams per day of doxycycline for 30 months. Another group of women with similar symptoms were given sugar pills (placebo) to take every day. The patients' pain was assessed at each visit, and x-rays were taken at the beginning and the end of the study. At the end of 30 months, the women who were treated with doxycycline were compared with those who took sugar pills. The results showed that women who took the doxycycline had less pain and less cartilage degradation, as compared to the women who took the sugar pills.

This study is encouraging, but because of several limitations in its design, we cannot say for sure that everyone with OA should start taking doxycycline. For example, the study included only middle-aged women, which begs the question, "Would doxycycline also work in men?" Additionally, the study examined a relatively small number of people (431) and evaluated them over a relatively short period of time. Would the results have been better or worse if the doxycycline therapy was continued? Experts have suggested that before doxycycline can be recommended as a treatment, larger studies must be done. The populations of the studies should include men and women as well as people from a variety of ethnic backgrounds. Until this kind of research is carried out, doxycycline should not be routinely prescribed for people with OA.

93. Can my osteoarthritis symptoms be improved with surgery?

Many surgical interventions can provide relief of OA-related symptoms. They range from office procedures that your rheumatologist can do under local anesthesia to major surgery performed by orthopedic surgery specialists that requires you to be hospitalized. These procedures include the injection of hyaluronic acid, steroids, or even new cartilage cells (chondrocytes) into the joint; arthroscopic procedures; and total joint replacement. The type of procedure that you might need depends on many factors, including your symptoms, the amount of disability you have, your general health status, and the skills and training of your orthopedic surgeon.

If you have OA of any joint that has progressed to the point it limits your ability to function or enjoy life, then you should consider surgery. For example, if you have hip or knee pain that cannot be controlled with medication or if your joint is so degenerated by OA that it no longer functions, then surgery may offer significant relief of pain and improvement in function.

The ultimate outcome of most orthopedic surgery depends on two factors: the skills of the surgeon and the willingness and ability of the patient to participate in a rehabilitation program for weeks or months after the procedure.

Unlike other types of surgery (for example, having your appendix removed), orthopedic surgery requires a greater investment of your time and effort after the procedure. The ultimate outcome of most orthopedic surgery depends on two factors: the skills of the surgeon and the willingness and ability of the patient to participate in a rehabilitation program for weeks or months after the procedure. Patients without the physical or mental ability to participate in a rigorous rehabilitation program are not considered good candidates for many procedures.

If you are considering surgery, discuss this issue with your primary care physician and your rheumatologist. They can advise you if you are a good candidate for a surgical procedure and explain what you can expect after the surgery.

94. Will my knee feel better if the doctor removes the fluid in it?

OA of the knees sometimes causes fluid to fill the joint, which causes swelling and pain. While this condition is commonly called "water on the knee," doctors may refer to the increased fluid more formally as a joint effusion. All of the movable (diarthrodial) joints in the body are surrounded by a layer of cells called the synovial membrane. This layer of cells normally produces a small amount of fluid, whose purpose is to lubricate the joints. OA can lead to irritation of the synovium and cause it to produce larger than normal amounts of joint fluid. This extra fluid may create visible swelling of the knee as well as increased pain and stiffness. If you develop swelling and pain in your knee, your doctor may suggest that you have the fluid removed in a procedure called an **arthrocentesis.**

Your physician may remove this fluid for two reasons. First, the procedure is diagnostic and can help your doctor determine what is causing the swelling. Second, the procedure itself may be therapeutic and help relieve the pain and stiffness of the knee.

The symptoms of swelling, pain, and stiffness in the knee can also be caused by processes other than OA, the most dangerous of which is an infection of the joint. If your doctor is not sure what is causing your knee pain and swelling, removing the joint fluid from the knee can help him or her to make a diagnosis of OA and exclude more serious problems such as joint infection (septic arthritis). Examination of the physical properties of the joint fluid, such as its color and clarity, and its white blood cell count can assist the physician in making these important determinations.

The removal of excess joint fluid can relieve pain, swelling, and stiffness, and improve the knee's range of motion and flexibility. Additionally, chronic knee effusions sometimes contribute to leg weakness. Removing extra joint fluid can be helpful in rebuilding quadriceps strength as well. The doctor may also inject corticosteroids ("cortisone") into the knee in an attempt to relieve arthritis symptoms. Sometimes this type of injection helps to prevent the joint fluid from reaccumulating. Corticosteroids can be injected approximately every three months, but if necessary the knee joint fluid can be drained more frequently.

Before performing an arthrocentesis, your doctor will clean your knee and the surrounding area with an antiseptic soap.

Arthrocentesis

The removal of fluid from a joint; also called joint aspiration. In this procedure, a sterile needle and syringe are used to drain fluid from a joint that is inflamed or infected.

Treatment of Ostheoarthritis

Next, the doctor will inject a medication, such as lidocaine, into the skin to numb the area. Finally, he or she will use a hypodermic needle to draw off the fluid. In experienced hands, this procedure does not cause much discomfort and usually takes five to ten minutes. You do not need to do any special preparation before this procedure, and you will usually feel better immediately.

95. Will arthroscopy help the pain in my knees?

Arthroscopy is a form of minimally invasive surgery that is performed on joints that have been injured through accident or disease. Arthroscopic procedures can be performed without opening the joint. These types of procedures have a lower risk of surgical complications than more invasive surgeries, reduce the amount of time you must spend in the hospital, and are associated with a quicker return to normal activity.

In arthroscopy, a specially trained surgeon passes a tube, known as an arthroscope, into the joint. The arthroscope contains both a light and a camera. It allows the surgeon to visualize structures inside the joint through a very small hole in the skin. Using another small hole, the surgeon can insert surgical instruments into the joint to repair injured structures. Sometimes a third incision is made so that the surgeon can insert additional surgical instruments or remove pieces of cartilage or bone that are causing pain and inflammation.

Tidal lavage

A treatment for osteoarthritis of the knee in which a saline solution is repeatedly injected, then withdrawn from the joint space to remove debris from the joint and help break up the synovial membrane, which has adhered to itself.

More than 500,000 arthroscopic procedures are performed each year in the United States. Approximately half of those patients report an improvement in pain and function after undergoing this type of surgery. The most common joint that arthroscopy is used on is the knee, and the most commonly performed arthroscopic procedures are tidal lavage and chondroplasty.

In **tidal lavage,** the surgeon removes small pieces of cartilage and other debris from the inside of the joint. After anesthetizing the patient, the surgeon injects sterile salt water into the joint several times. This fluid is allowed to wash out of another small hole in the joint. Many patients experience decreased pain and increased function following this procedure, with the improvements lasting several weeks or months.

In chondroplasty, the surgeon removes damaged cartilage from the joint and replaces it with new cartilage. The surgeon shaves off damaged cartilage from the inside of the joint and then removes some healthy cartilage from a part of the joint that does not bear weight or come in contact with other bones. The healthy cartilage is sent to a laboratory, which removes the healthy cartilage cells (called chondrocytes) from the cartilage. These new chondrocytes are placed back in the joint during a second surgical procedure. Some patients experience improvement in pain and function in their joints after this procedure. Chondroplasty is currently recommended for younger patients with joint injuries who want to prevent OA by repairing defective joint surfaces.

A study conducted in 2002 examined the effectiveness of arthroscopy in patients with OA of the knees. In half of the patients, an actual arthroscopic procedure was performed. In the other half, incisions were made in the skin of the knees of the anesthetized patients to make them think they had undergone surgery. When the physicians examined the patients and followed their progress over two years, they discovered that arthroscopic knee surgery was no more effective than sham surgery for relief of pain or stiffness from OA.

While this study doesn't mean that arthroscopy does not offer any benefit to any patient, its results should prompt debate on which procedure to perform and who is most likely to benefit. If you are considering arthroscopic surgery, discuss the likely risks and benefits with your rheumatologist and your orthopedist. Acting collaboratively, you should decide whether you are the best candidate for this procedure.

Treatment of Ostheoarthritis

96. Is joint replacement an option for the treatment of osteoarthritis symptoms?

Currently, medical science provides no cure for OA. Nevertheless, many therapies can reduce OA-related pain and increase joint function, including anti-inflammatory agents, painkillers, physical therapy, braces, orthotics, and lifestyle changes. All of these measures have been shown to reduce the symptoms of the disease. However, when these conservative treatments no longer provide relief, surgery is an option. This includes joint replacement surgery.

When conservative treatments for osteoarthritis no longer provide relief, surgery—including joint replacement—is an option.

The replacement of a natural joint with an artificial joint (i.e., prosthesis) is carried out through a surgical procedure called an arthroplasty. The two most commonly performed joint replacement procedures are hip and knee arthroplasties. Both are very successful procedures and are associated with high rates of patient satisfaction. They are by no means the only joint replacement procedures, however: Shoulder, elbow, wrist, and finger joints can also be replaced.

Not every person with an arthritic joint is a candidate for joint replacement. Joint replacement surgery is indicated for people who are in pain and have significant limitations of movement in the affected joint. These patients have usually failed to respond the more conservative treatment options. Even if a person meets all of these criteria, however, surgery may not be the most appropriate option. If the patient has other conditions that would increase the risk of complications or of prosthetic failure or that would render the individual unable to participate in a rigorous rehabilitation program, then he or she is unlikely to be considered for this type of surgery. For example, people with severe neurological, intellectual, or psychiatric impairment would not be able to participate in rehabilitation, nor would patients with severe heart or lung conditions. People with severe osteoporosis or obesity would also be at high risk for a failure of the prosthesis. Those with blood clotting disorders could be at excessive risk of pulmonary embolism (blood clots in the lung), strokes, or bleeding after surgery.

The timing of the surgery is important. For example, studies suggest that if a joint replacement is delayed too long, patients may become too debilitated to participate in their physical therapy after surgery. If a young person needs a joint replacement, his or her orthopedist will delay this surgery for as long as possible, because the implanted prosthesis will wear out. Thus a younger patient may eventually require one or more additional replacements in the future. Ideally, as surgical techniques and materials science improve over time, newer prostheses will be more durable and will require fewer replacements.

97. Can acupuncture improve my osteoarthritis–related pain?

Acupuncture is a branch of traditional Chinese medicine. It is based on the premise that the healthy body circulates an energy known as qi or chi. This energy circulates between the vital organs along channels or meridians. Blockages in these meridians result in an imbalance of qi, which results in disease. The traditional acupuncturist seeks to find the source of the imbalance and correct it by applying needles to various points along the meridians, called acupoints. More modern acupuncturists may employ other modalities to "unblock" the meridians, such as electricity, heat, pressure, and even laser light.

Numerous studies have examined the use of acupuncture in patients with OA. Recently, scientists at the U.S. National Health Service (NHS), a part of the U.S. Department of Health and Human Services, reviewed all of the available studies on the use of acupuncture for the treatment of OA. These researchers noted that the results of these studies were often confounded by small patient populations, variations in acupuncture technique, and the difficulty associated with finding an adequate "placebo" or sham procedure with which to compare the acupuncture. Nevertheless, they noted that most of these studies did not find a benefit for acupuncture when compared to sham acupuncture. They concluded that while the evidence is not sufficient to justify acupuncture as first-line treatment, it was probably sufficient to justify its use as a second- or third-line treatment. In addition, the authors suggested that the most appropriate candidate for acupuncture was a person who was not responding to conventional management, not tolerating medication, or experiencing recurrent pain.

Acupuncture is not without its downside. It is associated with some serious adverse events, including transmission of infectious disease, lung puncture (pneumothorax), other problems associated with organ punctures, spinal injuries, bleeding around the heart (cardiac tamponade), and broken needles left in the skin or other organs. Minor adverse events can include needles forgotten by the acupuncturist, worsening of pain and stiffness, minor bleeding, bruising, fatigue, sweating, severe nausea, fainting, and headache. The risk of adverse events tends to vary based on the practitioner's level of competence and training.

98. Is water therapy effective in the treatment of osteoarthritis-related pain and stiffness?

Water therapy, also known as pool therapy, aqua therapy, or hydrotherapy, can be effective in reducing the symptoms of OA. In particular, it can be a soothing way to stretch your muscles and reduce the pain from the impact of exercise done on land.

A heated pool is a great environment for exercise. It major advantage over land-based exercise is the heat and buoyancy provided by the water.

The heat of a warmed pool relaxes tired muscles and reduces aches and pains, which in turn allows for longer and less painful exercise sessions. The ideal temperature for water exercises is 83 to 88 degrees Fahrenheit. If the water is cooler, it does not relax the muscles as well. If the water temperature is higher, you can easily overheat while exercising.

Buoyancy is the tendency for a body to float in a liquid. It counteracts the press of gravity. For example, if you stand up to your neck in water, your feet support only 10% of your body weight; the water supports the rest. Someone standing up to his waist in water supports only 50% of his body weight. Reduced weight bearing reduces the stress across the joints, which in turn reduces the pain associated with OA and allows for longer and more vigorous exercise. This type of exercise is particularly helpful to patients with OA in the spine, hips, and knees, for whom almost any other exercise is too painful to tolerate.

Pools are not just for swimming, of course. Numerous forms of exercises can be practiced in the pool. Unlike similar exercises performed on land, exercises in the pool take advantage of both the buoyancy and the gentle resistance of the water against arms and legs. Types of exercises practiced in pools include the following:

- *Water aerobics*—including calisthenics, running in place, water walking, or using cross-country skiing movements in a shallow pool.
- *Stretching*—including stretching the lower back, hamstrings, and calf muscles; touching the toes; and slowly raising the knees to the chest.
- *Strengthening*—including muscle-building exercises, the use of foam barbells or hand paddles to complete bicep curls, and lateral side raises that work against water resistance.
- *Ai chi*—a form of tai chi that was developed specifically for exercise in pools. Its slow, gentle, and rhythmic movements develop strength, balance, and joint flexibility.

As with any exercise program, you should start by visiting your doctor and making sure that you can tolerate the exercise without undue risk before you begin any type of water therapy.

99. Can cartilage be replaced?

Surgery for the repair of knee cartilage is commonplace today. It involves removing loose cartilage and smoothing the surface of existing cartilage. But what if cartilage is missing—can a defect in the surface of the cartilage be repaired in such a case? In fact, surgeons in Sweden began performing this type of surgery more than a decade ago. They removed small, matchstick-shaped pieces of cartilage from areas of the knee that did not bear weight and inserted them into areas on the weight-bearing surface where cartilage was missing. This technique worked reasonably well—but what if you did not have enough cartilage tissue to graft?

To address this issue, scientists developed a process for harvesting cartilage cells, growing them outside the body, and then replacing them into a damaged joint. The company that initially developed this laboratory technique, Genzyme Biosurgery, calls its product Carticel. More generally, the surgical procedure of harvesting, culturing, and replacing the cells is called autologous chondrocyte implantation (ACI) or autologous chondrocyte transfer (ACT). The word "autologous" means that the person uses his or her own cartilage cells to grow new cells; that is, the cells are not donated by another person.

The ACI technique involves a two-step surgical procedure. In the first surgery, the surgeon removes a small amount of cartilage tissue. The cells in this tissue (chondrocytes) are then brought to a lab, where they can be grown and the population of cells can be multiplied. When there are a sufficient number of cells (usually after a few weeks), a second surgery is performed, in which the cells are placed in the cartilage defect in the joint. Over time, these cells develop into cartilage and significantly improve the function of the joint.

The disadvantages of this procedure include its high cost and the length of the rehabilitation following the surgery, which can take months of exercise and crutch walking. This technique has been approved by the FDA for people who have experienced cartilage-related injuries from sports or other accidents, but it is not an approved therapy for people with OA.

Research continues on ways to employ ACI to help patients with OA. For example, tissue engineers are working on techniques to grow larger amounts of chondrocytes in a customized mold that has the same size and shape as the damaged joint surface. It is hoped that these cells will be able to replace all of the cartilage in a joint and that their implantation will not require the prolonged rehabilitation period needed today.

100. What are other resources for people with arthritis?

The following websites, books, and magazines may be helpful to patients with arthritis.

Organizations

American College of Rheumatology
1800 Century Place
Suite 250
Atlanta, GA 30345-4300
Phone: 404-633-3777
Fax: 404-633-1870
http://www.rheumatology.org
The American College of Rheumatology is an organization of and for physicians, health professionals, and scientists. Its goal is to advance rheumatology through programs of education, research, advocacy, and practice support that foster

excellence in the care of people with arthritis and rheumatic and musculoskeletal diseases.

Arthritis Foundation
P.O. Box 7669
Atlanta, GA 30357-0669
Phone: 800-568-4045
http://www.arthritis.org
Currently this website has a link with which you can obtain a free kit on rheumatoid arthritis. "It is designed to give you tools and tips to better communicate with your rheumatologist about your symptoms and how to get the most from your office visits." The Arthritis Foundation provides lots of information on arthritis, and a long list of useful links to other websites.

Arthritis National Research Foundation
200 Oceangate
Suite 830
Long Beach, CA 90802
Phone: 800-588-2873
Fax: 562-983-1410
E-mail: anrf@ix.netcom.com
The Arthritis National Research Foundation offers funding to promising young scientists at the beginning of their research careers to pursue cutting-edge projects for the treatment, cure, and eventual end to the suffering of the more than 66 million Americans with arthritis and its related diseases.

Arthritis Research Institute of America
300 South Duncan Avenue
Suite 188
Clearwater, FL 33755
Phone: 727-461-4054
Fax: 727-449-9227
E-mail: info@preventarthritis.org

The Arthritis Research Institute of America is a national nonprofit, public charity with tax-exempt status. The institute was founded on the premise that important areas of arthritis research needed to be addressed, that the urgency of those needs was increasing, and that the institute could provide effective, innovative, and cost-effective ways to meet those needs. The institute's mission is to identify the causes, seek preventive measures, and find a cure for osteoarthritis. The nature of the research is primarily community-based studies as well as clinical studies.

Arthritis Society (National Office)
393 University Avenue, Suite 1700
Toronto, Ontario M5G 1E6
Canada
Phone: 416-979-7228
Fax: 416-979-8366
E-mail: info@arthritis.ca

Websites

Johns Hopkins Arthritis Center
www.hopkins-arthritis.som.jhmi.edu/index.html
The Johns Hopkins Arthritis Center is a very useful source of scientific updates in the field of arthritis. Its website is a great resource for both doctors and patients. The site includes an entire section on rheumatoid arthritis. You can also download a rheumatoid arthritis activity minder—a tool for monitoring disease activity so you can objectively keep track of your course and have better communication with your doctor.

MayoClinic.com
http://www.mayoclinic.com/health/rheumatoid-arthritis/DS00020/DSECTION=8&
This is a great website from the people at the Mayo Clinic. It has excellent information about rheumatoid arthritis and its treatments.

Medicinenet

http://www.medicinenet.com/rheumatoid_arthritis/article
.htm
MedicineNet.com is an online, healthcare media publishing company. Its website provides authoritative medical information on rheumatoid arthritis and other topics for consumers.

Medline Plus

www.nlm.nih.gov/medlineplus/medlineplus.html
Medline plus is a project of the National Library of Medicine. This website provides useful information on almost any topic and includes very useful information on medications.

Rituxan.com

http://www.rituxan.com/ra/index.jsp
This website is sponsored by Genentech, the makers of Rituxan (rituximab.) It provides information about rheumatoid arthritis, and questions and answers about Rituxan.

Magazines

Arthritis Today
This magazine, which is available from the Arthritis Foundation, contains useful articles on how to live with rheumatoid arthritis and updates medications and new treatments.

Audacity Magazine
This news and entertainment magazine is geared toward the disability community in the United States and the world.

Books

The Arthritis Foundation's Guide to Good Living with Rheumatoid Arthritis, third edition
By Dorothy Foltz-Gray
Available in bookstores and from online retailers.
A plain-English guide to rheumatoid arthritis, its symp-

toms, and its treatments. This book is sponsored by the
Arthritis Foundation.

The Arthritis Helpbook
By Kate Lorig and James Fries
Available from the Arthritis Foundation or from booksellers.
This is a very helpful book with useful tips for learning to
live with arthritis.

The First Year—Rheumatoid Arthritis: An Essential Guide for
the Newly Diagnosed (First Year)
By M. E. A. McNeil
Available in bookstores and from online retailers.
A first-person account of the author's struggle with rheumatoid arthritis as well as her insights into the disease and
its treatments.

Treatment of Ostheoarthritis

Glossary

A

Arthritis: Inflammation of a joint, usually accompanied by pain, swelling, and stiffness.

Anemia: The condition of having less than the normal number of red blood cells or less than the normal quantity of hemoglobin in the blood. Anemia is associated with rheumatoid arthritis and other chronic diseases. It is a complication of the use of nonsteroidal anti-inflammatory drugs (NSAIDs).

Ankylosing: Crooked or bent; refers to stiffening of the joint.

Antibodies: Proteins produced by white blood cells to fight foreign proteins, viruses, bacteria, and other unfamiliar invaders.

Antigen: A foreign protein or carbohydrate complex that causes an immune response.

Antimalarials: Drugs normally used to treat malaria but that are sometimes effective in the treatment of rheumatoid arthritis. The most commonly used antimalarial is hydroxychloroquine sulfate (Plaquenil).

Antinuclear antibody (ANA): An unusual antibody that is directed against structures within the nucleus of the human cell. ANAs are found in patients whose immune systems are predisposed to cause inflammation against their own body tissues.

Arthr-: A prefix meaning "joint."

Arthrocentesis: The removal of fluid from a joint; also called joint aspiration. In this procedure, a sterile needle and syringe are used to drain fluid from a joint that is inflamed or infected.

Arthroplasty: Implantation of a mechanical joint to replace a diseased or damaged joint; also called total joint replacement surgery.

Arthroscopy: A diagnostic and surgical technique that uses a thin tube with a light and a tiny video camera at one end to view the inside of a joint.

Articular cartilage: Tough, rubbery tissue that forms the surface of bones within joints.

Autoimmune disease: A disease that arises when an individual's immune system reacts against his or her own organs and tissues.

Autoimmune disorder: A disorder that results when the body's tissues are attacked by its own immune system. Rheumatoid arthritis and systemic lupus erythematosus are examples of autoimmune disorders.

B

Bisphosphonate: One of a class of drugs used to maintain or improve bone density.

Bone remodeling: A cyclical process by which bone maintains a dynamic steady state through resorption and formation of a small amount of bone at the same site. Bone remodeling can occur as a result of joint disease.

Bouchard's nodes: Knobby over-growths of the middle joint of the fingers in people with osteoarthritis.

C

Chondrocyte: A cartilage cell.

Chondroitin sulfate: A sugar-based material that is present in cartilage. Chondroitin is a popular dietary supplement that is thought to improve the joint symptoms of osteoarthritis.

Chronic: Lasting for a long time. The word comes from the Greek *chronos,* which means "time."

Citrulline antibody: An antibody directed against an unusual amino acid called citrulline. Citrulline is not normally present in peptides or pro-teins in the body. The presence of high amounts of the citrulline antibody in the bloodstream suggests that the person is suffering from rheumatoid arthritis.

Collagen: The major protein of con-nective tissue, cartilage, and bone.

Collagen: The main structural protein in connective tissue.

Complete blood count (CBC): A test that gives information about the cells in a person's blood.

Conjunctivitis: An inflammation of the outer membrane of the eye.

Connective tissue: The material that holds various body structures together. Cartilage, tendons, ligaments, and blood vessels are composed entirely of connective tissue.

Coronary artery disease: A narrowing of the coronary arteries that results in inadequate blood flow to the heart.

Corticosteroids: Any of the steroid hormones made by the cortex (outer layer) of the adrenal gland; also called cortisol and steroids. These potent drugs are used to reduce the pain and inflammation associated with rheuma-toid arthritis and other autoimmune disorders.

C-reactive protein (CRP): A type of protein that is made in the liver. The amount of CRP rises in the blood in conjunction with the inflammation produced by certain conditions.

Crepitus: A crackling sound or grat-ing sensation in a joint, caused by swollen synovium or bone surface rubbing together.

D

Degenerative joint disease (DJD): Joint destruction that occurs over a long period of time. This term is used synonymously with the term "osteoarthritis."

Diagnosis: The identification of an illness after review of the patient's clinical history, physical exam, and laboratory tests.

Disease-modifying antirheumatic drugs (DMARDs): A class of medications that are used to treat arthritis and other rheumatic conditions. Examples include methotrexate, leflunomide, and sulfasalizine.

E

Enzyme: Any protein that regulates chemical changes in other substances.

Erosion: From the Latin *erodere*, meaning "to eat away"; an eating away of a surface. Erosion of the bone surface of joints is a common feature of many types of arthritis.

Erythrocyte sedimentation rate (ESR): A diagnostic test for inflammatory diseases that measures the rate at which red blood cells settle out from a well-mixed specimen of blood.

F

Fatigue: A condition characterized by a lessened capacity for work and reduced efficiency of accomplishment, usually accompanied by a feeling of weariness and tiredness.

Flare: The reappearance or worsening of arthritic symptoms.

G

Glucosamine: An amino sugar produced by the body that is found in cartilage. Glucosamine is a popular dietary supplement and is thought to improve the joints symptoms of osteoarthritis.

Gout: A disease characterized by increased blood levels of uric acid; it produces pain and inflammation in the joints, particularly in the foot, ankle, and knee.

H

Heberden's nodes: Knobby overgrowths of the joint nearest the fingertips in patients with osteoarthritis.

I

Immunosuppressive therapy (immunosuppressant): An agent capable of suppressing the immune response. Such medications increase a person's risk for infection and malignancy.

Inflammation: A response to injury or foreign invasion that is designed to protect the body. Its symptoms include heat, redness, swelling, and pain.

L

Ligament: A thin layer of connective tissue that holds the tooth in its socket, and acts as a cushion between tooth and bone.

Lymphoma: A cancer of the lymphoid tissue.

M

Magnetic resonance imaging (MRI): A diagnostic technique in which radio waves generated in a strong magnetic field are used to provide information about the hydrogen atoms in different tissues within the body. A computer then uses this information to produce images of the tissues in many different planes.

N

Nonsteroidal anti-inflammatory drugs (NSAIDs): Medications that relieve joint pain and stiffness by reducing inflammation. Examples include aspirin and ibuprofen.

O

Osteoarthritis (OA): A type of arthritis characterized by pain and stiffness in the joints, such as those in the hands, hips, knees, spine, or feet; it is caused by the breakdown of cartilage.

Osteophyte: An outgrowth of bone.

Osteoporosis: A disease characterized by the thinning of the bones with a reduction in bone mass owing to depletion of calcium and bone protein. Osteoporosis predisposes a person to fractures.

P

Platelet: An irregular, disc-shaped element in the blood that assists in blood clotting.

Primary osteoarthritis: The gradual breakdown of cartilage that occurs with age and is caused by stress on a joint.

Progressive: An adjective applied to many diseases; it suggests an increase in scope or severity of disease.

Prostaglandins: Chemicals that produce pain and inflammation.

R

Range of motion (ROM): Measurement of joint movement angle, which may be restricted due to inflammation.

Remission: A period in the course of a disease during which symptoms of a disease diminish or disappear.

Rheumatic disease: Any one of more than 100 disorders that cause inflammation in connective tissues.

Rheumatoid arthritis (RA): A chronic autoimmune disease characterized by pain, stiffness, inflammation, swelling, and sometimes destruction of joints.

Rheumatoid factor (RF): An antibody found in about 85% of people with rheumatoid arthritis; it also appears in other diseases and is sometimes found in healthy people.

Rheumatoid nodules: Firm, nonpainful lumps in the skin of patients with rheumatoid arthritis. These nodules tend to occur at pressure points of the body—most commonly, the elbows. They are a sign of long-standing rheumatoid arthritis.

Rheumatologist: A physician who specializes in the treatment of diseases of the joints and connective tissue.

Rheumatology: The branch of medicine devoted to the study and treatment of connective tissue diseases.

S

Secondary osteoarthritis: Osteoarthritis that results from trauma to the joint or from chronic joint injury due to another type of arthritis, such as rheumatoid arthritis.

Septic arthritis: Arthritis caused by invading microorganisms.

Side effects: A term associated with medical treatments; problems that occur when a treatment has consequences that go beyond the desired effect, or when the patient develops problems that occur in addition to the desired therapeutic effect.

Synovectomy: Removal of the synovial membrane of a joint.

Synovial fluid: A lubricating fluid secreted by the synovial membrane.

Synovial membrane: Connective tissue that lines the cavity of a joint and produces synovial fluid.

Synovitis: Inflammation of the synovium.

Systemic: An adjective used in medicine to indicate something that affects the entire body, rather than a single part or organ.

T

Tidal lavage: A treatment for osteoarthritis of the knee in which a saline solution is repeatedly injected, then withdrawn from the joint space to remove debris from the joint and help break up the synovial membrane, which has adhered to itself.

Total hip replacement: A type of surgery in which the diseased ball and socket of the hip joint are completely removed and replaced with artificial materials. Also called a hip arthroplasty.

Total knee replacement: A surgical procedure in which damaged parts of the knee joint are replaced with artificial parts, which are usually made of plastic and steel.

Tumor necrosis factor (TNF): A protein that plays an early and major role in the rheumatic disease process.

V

Vasculitis: Inflammation of blood vessels. 9

Viscosupplementation: A treatment option for people with osteoarthritis of the knee that involves the injection of hyaluronan, a natural component of synovial fluid, directly into the knee joint.

Vitamin D: A fat-soluble vitamin that causes the intestines to increase absorption and metabolism of the minerals calcium and phosphorus (the building blocks of bone).

Index